Cambridge Elements ≡

Elements of Genetics in Epilepsy
edited by
Annapurna H. Poduri
Boston Children's Hospital and Harvard Medical School
Alfred L. George, Jr.
Northwestern University Feinberg School of Medicine
Erin L. Heinzen
University of North Carolina, Chapel Hill
Sara James
KCNQ2 Cure Alliance and Genetic Epilepsy Team Australia

KCNQ2- AND *KCNQ3-* ASSOCIATED EPILEPSY

Edited by

Sarah Weckhuysen
Antwerp University Hospital

Alfred L. George, Jr.
Northwestern University Feinberg School of Medicine

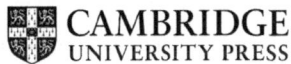

CAMBRIDGE
UNIVERSITY PRESS

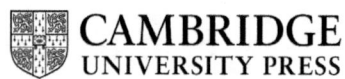

CAMBRIDGE
UNIVERSITY PRESS

Shaftesbury Road, Cambridge CB2 8EA, United Kingdom

One Liberty Plaza, 20th Floor, New York, NY 10006, USA

477 Williamstown Road, Port Melbourne, VIC 3207, Australia

314–321, 3rd Floor, Plot 3, Splendor Forum, Jasola District Centre,
New Delhi – 110025, India

103 Penang Road, #05–06/07, Visioncrest Commercial, Singapore 238467

Cambridge University Press is part of Cambridge University Press & Assessment,
a department of the University of Cambridge.

We share the University's mission to contribute to society through the pursuit of
education, learning and research at the highest international levels of excellence.

www.cambridge.org
Information on this title: www.cambridge.org/9781009278263

DOI: 10.1017/9781009278270

A catalogue record for this publication is available from the British Library.

ISBN 978-1-009-27826-3 Paperback
ISSN 2633-2086 (online)
ISSN 2633-2078 (print)

Additional resources for this publication at www.cambridge.org/weckhuysen-george

Cambridge University Press & Assessment has no responsibility for the persistence
or accuracy of URLs for external or third-party internet websites referred to in this
publication and does not guarantee that any content on such websites is, or will
remain, accurate or appropriate.

Every effort has been made in preparing this Element to provide accurate and up-to-date
information which is in accord with accepted standards and practice at the time of publication.
Although case histories are drawn from actual cases, every effort has been made to disguise the
identities of the individuals involved. Nevertheless, the authors, editors and publishers can make
no warranties that the information contained herein is totally free from error, not least because
clinical standards are constantly changing through research and regulation. The authors, editors
and publishers therefore disclaim all liability for direct or consequential damages resulting from
the use of material contained in this Element. Readers are strongly advised to pay careful attention
to information provided by the manufacturer of any drugs or equipment that they plan to use.

KCNQ2- and *KCNQ3*-Associated Epilepsy

Elements of Genetics in Epilepsy

DOI: 10.1017/9781009278270
First published online: November 2022

Sarah Weckhuysen
Antwerp University Hospital

Alfred L. George, Jr.
Northwestern University Feinberg School of Medicine

Author for correspondence: Alfred L. George, Jr., al.george@northwestern.edu

Abstract: *KCNQ2* and *KCNQ3* encode subunits ($K_V7.2$, $K_V7.3$) that combine to form a voltage-gated potassium ion (K^+) channel responsible for generating an ionic current (M-current) important for controlling activity in the nervous system. Pathogenic variants in both genes are associated with a spectrum of genetic neurological disorders that feature epilepsy of variable severity and can be accompanied by debilitating impaired neurodevelopment. These two genes were among the first discovered causes of monogenic epilepsy, and are frequently identified in persons with early-life epilepsy. This Element provides a comprehensive review of the clinical features, genetic basis, pathophysiology, pharmacology, and treatment of these prototypical neurological disorders, accompanied by perspectives shared by affected families and scientists who have made seminal contributions to the field. This title is also available as Open Access on Cambridge Core.

Keywords: epilepsy, potassium channel, neonatal seizures, retigabine, M-current

ISBNs: 9781009278263 (PB), 9781009278270 (OC)
ISSNs: 2633-2086 (online), 2633-2078 (print)

Contents

Contributors

Maria Roberta Cilio, M.D.
Catholic University of Louvain
Alfred L. George, Jr., M.D.
Northwestern University Feinberg School of Medicine
Sara James
KCNQ2 Cure Alliance
Caroline Loewy
KCNQ2 Cure Alliance
Tristan Sands, M.D., Ph.D.
Columbia University Irving Medical Center
Scotty Sims
KCNQ2 Cure Alliance
Maurizio Taglialatela, M.D., Ph.D.
University of Naples Federico II
Tammy N. Tsuchida, M.D., Ph.D.
George Washington University School of Medicine and Health Sciences
Anastasios Tzingounis, Ph.D.
University of Connecticut
Sarah Weckhuysen, M.D., Ph.D.
Antwerp University Hospital

Introduction

This is the first gene-focused Element of the Cambridge Elements Genetics in Epilepsy series launched in September 2021 [1]. The goal of this issue is to provide an in-depth, state-of-the-art review of clinical, genetic, basic science, and family perspectives on epilepsies associated with pathogenic variants in two genes, *KCNQ2* and *KCNQ3*, that encode key components of a vital neuronal potassium channel. In many respects, these two genes and the associated neurological disorders are prototypical of monogenic epilepsies. Indeed, *KCNQ2* and *KCNQ3* were among the earliest discoveries in the genetics of epilepsy [2,3], and are still frequently identified in early-life epilepsies [4]. The evolution of progress in understanding these disorders has been rapid and rewarding (**Fig. 1**). Because there are considerably more known cases with *KCNQ2* pathogenic variants, there is greater emphasis on this gene and its gene product – the potassium channel known as $K_V7.2$ or KCNQ2 (protein name is not italicized).

We hope this Element will provide opportunities for families, trainees, and healthcare professionals to learn about *KCNQ2*- and *KCNQ3*-associated epilepsy from multiple vantage points. There are detailed discussions of the clinical features, pathophysiology, pharmacology, genetics, and treatment. The Element begins with detailed perspectives from parents of children with these disorders, including findings from recent surveys, which were generated by a parent-led advocacy group (KCNQ2 Cure Alliance), designed to quantify seizure and nonseizure aspects of these disorders. This section is followed by an in-depth review of the neurophysiology, pathophysiology, and pharmacology of neuronal M-current generated by *KCNQ2/KCNQ3*-encoded potassium channel subunits. The last sections of this Element are devoted to descriptions of the clinical spectrum and treatment of *KCNQ2*- and *KCNQ3*-associated neurodevelopmental disorders.

In addition to the thorough and informative narrative, this Element of Genetics in Epilepsy is enlivened by unique video content including interviews with Professor David Brown on the discovery of the neuronal M-current (**Video 3**), with Dr. Nanda Singh on the genetic links of *KCNQ2* and *KCNQ3* with epilepsy (**Video 4**), and with Professor Anne Berg on the features and natural history of *KCNQ2*-associated epilepsy (**Video 1**). This Element also presents five parents of children with *KCNQ2* developmental and epileptic encephalopathy who share their stories of life with this disorder (**Video 2**), and a panel discussion of scientists on their motivations to investigate the biology of *KCNQ2* and *KCNQ3* (**Video 5**). Finally, **Video 6** and **Video 7** show the typical seizure semiology in newborns with *KCNQ2*-associated epilepsy.

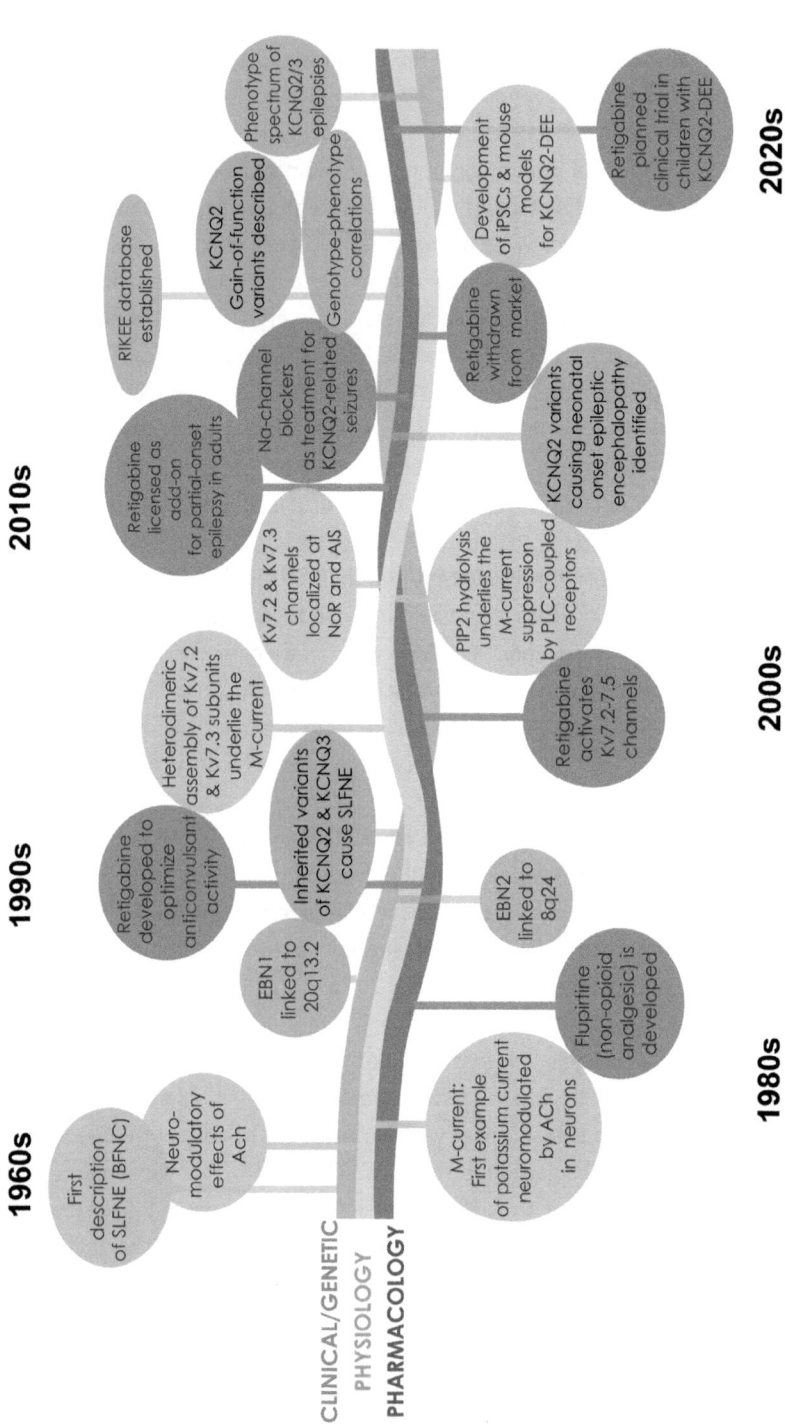

Figure 1 Timeline of discoveries related to *KCNQ2*- and *KCNQ3*-associated epilepsy. Major discoveries regarding clinical and genetic advances, physiology, and pharmacology are illustrated by different colored lines and text boxes.

We are grateful for the contributions by the many coauthors of this issue, and for the contributors of the video content, especially Sara James who conducted most of the interviews remotely from her home in Australia. We also acknowledge the artistry of Rebecca Oramas for drawing Figures 1, 11 and 12, and the team of Stephanie McCormack, Enrique Rojas, and Abbie Van Nuland for helping Dr. Berg produce infographics from the KCNQ2 Natural History Study (Figures 2–10). Finally, we appreciate the editorial assistance of Shaye Moore in proofreading the manuscript and transcribing the videos. This was a team effort that we hope provides inspiration to future clinicians, researchers, and patient advocates. We hope you enjoy learning about these two important epilepsy genes.

Patient, Family, and Foundation Perspectives

KCNQ2 developmental and epileptic encephalopathy (KCNQ2-DEE) is a multifaceted genetic disorder that has significant impact on both the individual and the family. Its classification as a genetic *epilepsy* focuses attention on seizures, which occur in the majority of individuals with KCNQ2-DEE. But seizures may decline in frequency or disappear altogether as the child ages, and many with KCNQ2-DEE are able to achieve some degree of seizure control with medication. Not everyone who suffers from KCNQ2-DEE has clinically recognized seizures, and it is important to note that seizures are only a part of this complex condition. As families rapidly learn, the associated comorbidities, or *coexpressions* (term coined by Anne Berg, Ph.D.; see **Video 1**), can be most daunting and life-changing; people with KCNQ2-DEE also may have intellectual disability, impaired communication, compromised motor function, gastrointestinal dysfunction, and autism, among other difficulties.

KCNQ2 Cure Alliance Foundation

The KCNQ2 Cure Alliance Foundation[1] was founded in 2014 by a group of four parents determined to support research, improve understanding of this rare disorder, support those affected by KCNQ2-DEE, and work collaboratively to find a cure for this life-altering disease. From a simple Facebook post that

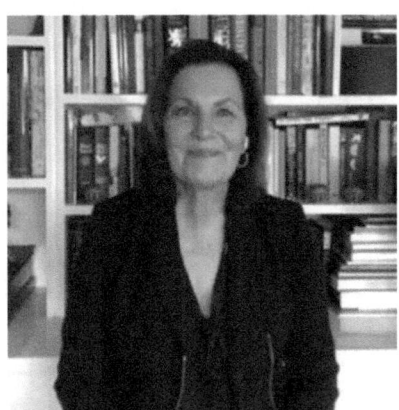
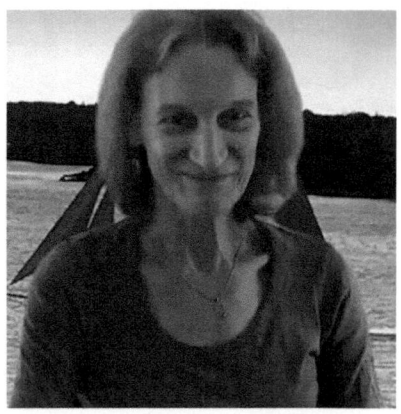

Sara James   Anne Berg, Ph.D.

Video 1 Anne Berg, Ph.D. (Professor, Northwestern University) discusses clinical coexpressions of KCNQ2-DEE and the KCNQ2 Natural History Study. A video transcript can be found in the Appendix. The video file is available at www.cambridge.org/weckhuysen-george

---

[1] www.kcnq2cure.org.

connected a handful of families, the Foundation's parent and caregiver support group has grown to more than 800 people from more than 60 countries. KCNQ2 Cure Alliance also collaborates with regional KCNQ2 organizations and foundations in Australia, France, Germany, Italy, and Spain, expanding the reach of the organization. In addition to its virtual presence, KCNQ2 Cure Alliance hosts family and professional summits, and advocates for research and development of new treatment options for KCNQ2-DEE. Despite all of these efforts, there are no approved treatments, and there are thousands more patients who remain undiagnosed and who have not yet been reached.

KCNQ2 Cure Alliance raises funds to support clinical and basic-science research conducted at internationally respected institutions. The Foundation leverages its fundraising efforts with grant support and collaborations with for-profit companies that have promising new ideas. Among these efforts, the Foundation has funded or helped to fund a natural history study and creation of mouse models and cell lines. The Foundation collaborates in the conduct of clinical trials, including a clinical trial of ezogabine.

KCNQ2 Cure Alliance funds more than scientific research. The Foundation also raises money to support education, advocacy, patient/family support, and awareness on the international, national, and local levels. Bringing families and scientists together is crucial. The Foundation's annual family and professional summit offers families the chance to meet others in the community, with travel scholarships available for families who would not otherwise be able to attend. The summit also allows scientists, clinicians, and those in the biopharmaceutical industry to connect and collaborate with each other, and with the patient community.

KCNQ2 Cure Alliance is proud to have an active parent community. Donations come from generous grandparents, parents, and friends, and from many others who have no personal connection to KCNQ2-DEE or genetic epilepsy. There are online campaigns, cocktail parties, t-shirt sales, holiday card sales, a virtual walk, and big events attended by hundreds of people such as the annual *KCNQ2 Cure New Horizons in Science Dinner* in Melbourne, Australia.

Groups like the KCNQ2 Cure Alliance have united the community, but part of what makes KCNQ2-DEE especially challenging is that there is a broad spectrum of phenotypes associated with hundreds of distinct *KCNQ2* variants. While patients share many features, each KCNQ2-DEE case is unique.

KCNQ2-DEE is underdiagnosed and there is often a long diagnostic journey. In recent years, rapid genetic testing has made it possible for some children to be diagnosed within days of birth. Others in the KCNQ2 community report receiving a diagnosis much later, including some in their fifth decade of life. Older patients who exhausted diagnostic efforts prior to the clinical description of KCNQ2-DEE and availability of genetic testing remain undiagnosed or misdiagnosed. The diagnostic delay is responsible for the skewed demographics of the patient population, with 63% of patients in the Natural History Study aged one to four years (**Fig. 2**).

There are advantages and disadvantages to both early and late diagnoses. Families whose newborn is diagnosed secure an answer and the ability to connect with other families in the KCNQ2 community. Hope comes to parents and caregivers from learning about the latest research, but also the burden of knowledge as they come to terms with the prognosis and the profound implications of what the future may hold.

Those who did not receive a diagnosis until later sometimes express relief that they did not appreciate the full extent of the disorder's potential complications. At the same time, they express frustration for having lived years without a complete or correct diagnosis. Many parents report a sense of relief to learn that their child has a *KCNQ2* pathogenic variant, which for most is de novo and not because of something they did. They express gratitude for the connection with other families who understand what they are going through.

> *The diagnosis of KCNQ2 has been … a weight off my mind. [Our daughter] was 25 when we got the diagnosis. [Her] disabilities have just been part of my life. A professor told us at 9 months old that she would never amount to anything in life and basically be a vegetable and if we wanted to walk away then and there, the hospital would arrange for her to go into care. We picked her up and I have fought for her for 31 years.*
>
> Mother of an adult daughter in the United Kingdom

KCNQ2 Cure Alliance recognizes the need to help families at every stage of their journey and is looking for new ways to support the increasing number of

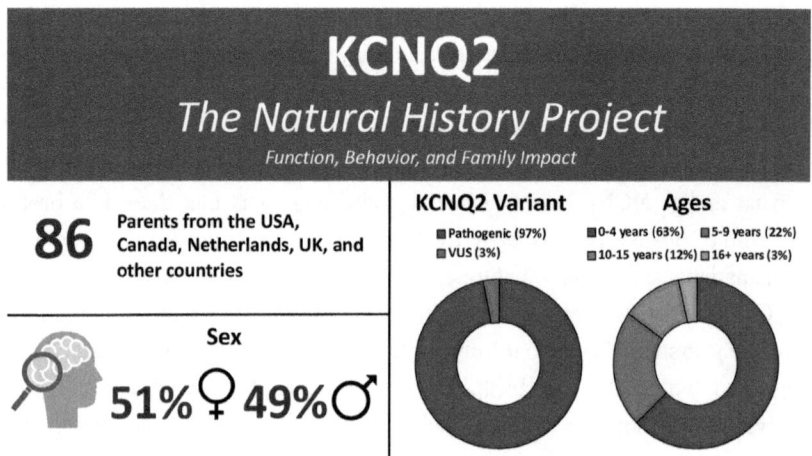

Figure 2 Summary of participants in the KCNQ2 Natural History Study.

families who receive an early diagnosis for their child as well as those with older children who are diagnosed late.

KCNQ2 "Coexpressions"

Anne T. Berg, Ph.D. (Northwestern University Feinberg School of Medicine) recognized the need to learn more about nonseizure aspects of KCNQ2-DEE. She created a detailed survey to identify the myriad ways KCNQ2-DEE can affect an individual (**Video 1**). Caregivers representing 86 patients ranging in age from birth to older than 16 years participated in the KCNQ2 Natural History Study (**Fig. 2**), and the results are published [5,6].

Most respondents (95%) report that first seizures occurred within the first month of life. Communication was one of the most commonly cited nonseizure concerns. Among parents surveyed, 73% of those with children older than four years reported that their child does not speak any words, and 66% responded that their child inconsistently or rarely communicates, even with people they know. Impaired mobility is also a common feature; nearly half of children older than four years report dependence on a wheeled mobility device. A similar proportion noted that their child is completely dependent on a caregiver for feeding. Approximately half also responded that their child suffers from non-seizure-related sleep disturbances. A majority of families report that their child suffers some sort of gastrointestinal difficulties, with 69% of respondents reporting that their children have constipation. More than a third of families (37% of respondents) said their children with KCNQ2-DEE also have a diagnosis of autism or have autistic features. Given these statistics, it is not surprising that 60% of parents reported moderate to severe fatigue.

To get a better picture of the myriad ways in which KCNQ2-DEE affects an individual and all of those who love and care for them, the KCNQ2 Cure Alliance conducted a survey of KCNQ2-DEE families. Specifically, members of the parent/caregiver support group were asked a series of questions related to various features of KCNQ2-DEE that had been highlighted in the KCNQ2 Natural History Study. Included in the survey were questionnaires about seizures, functional ability, activities of daily living, communication skills, gastrointestinal issues, behavior, sleep, autonomic nervous system dysfunction, what children enjoy, the overall impact of KCNQ2-DEE on the individual and the family, and if there were any silver linings.

Sixty-five families responded to the survey. Not every question is relevant to every family equally; consequently, some questions garnered more responses than others. Interestingly, all of the parents who completed the questionnaire were mothers. While KCNQ2-DEE is evenly distributed in the general population between boys and girls, nearly 60% of questionnaire respondents are the mothers of girls or women with KCNQ2-DEE. The age of those individuals ranged from 4 months to 37 years.

What follows is a summary of the results of the KCNQ2 Cure Alliance survey and the KCNQ2 Natural History Study. Note that parents often refer to the disease as "KCNQ2" rather than KCNQ2-DEE. Some of the responding parents are featured in **Video 2**.

Seizures are one of the few characteristics that affect nearly all of those diagnosed with KCNQ2-DEE (**Fig. 3**). Even so, the degree to which seizures impact the patient and their caregivers is highly variable. Among those participating in the KCNQ2 Cure survey, 60 parents reported seizures in their children, with 83% reporting that their child's seizures began in the first 72 hours of life. Intriguingly, 5% of parents reported that their child never had a clinically recognizable seizure. Many mothers believe their child had seizures in utero (60% of respondents).

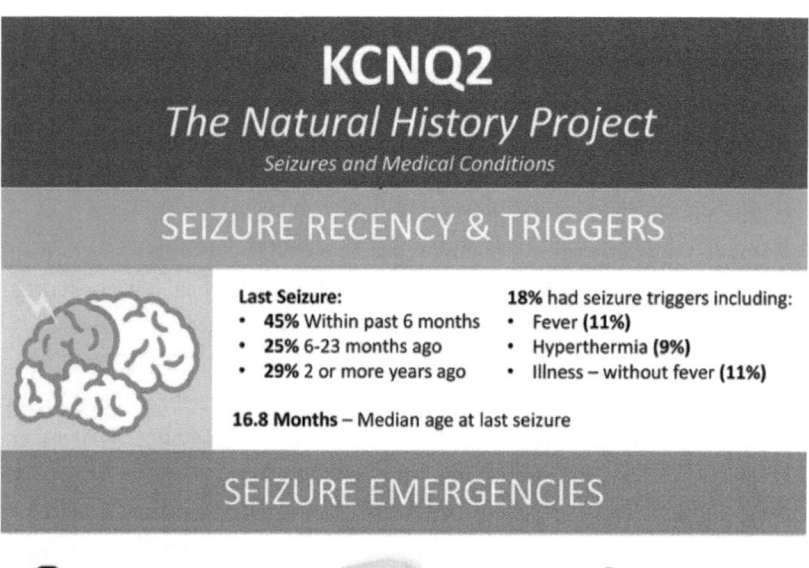
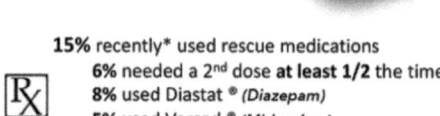

Figure 3 Summary of seizure data in the KCNQ2 Natural History Study.

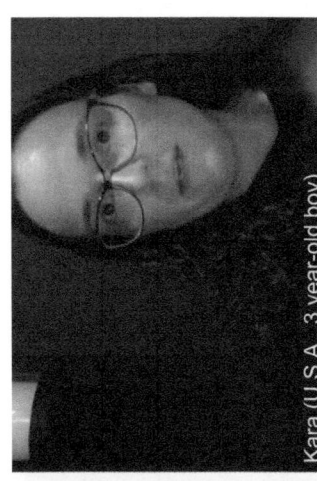

Kara (U.S.A., 3 year-old boy)

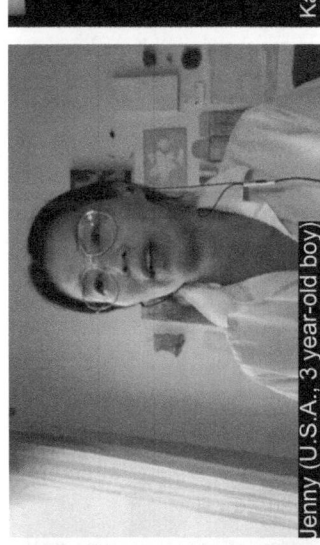

Jenny (U.S.A., 3 year-old boy)

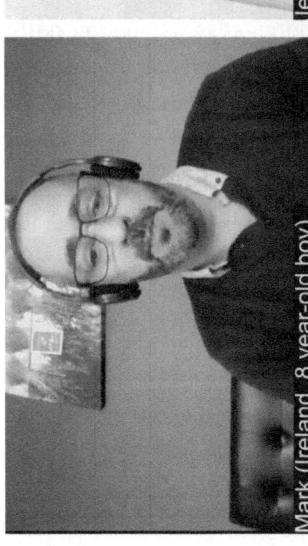

Mark (Ireland, 8 year-old boy)

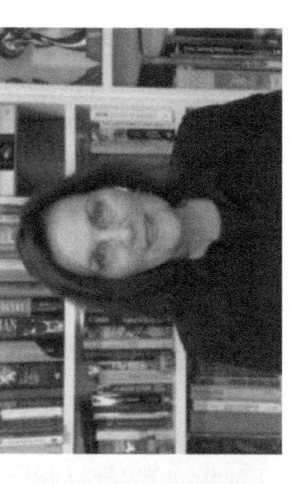

Claire (France, 6 year-old boy)

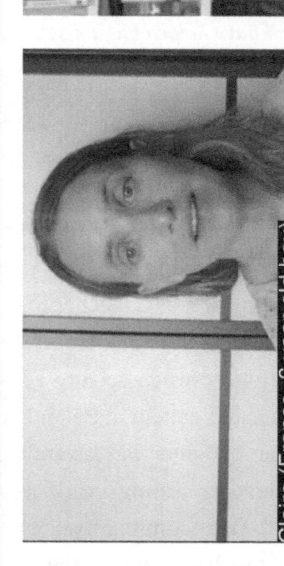

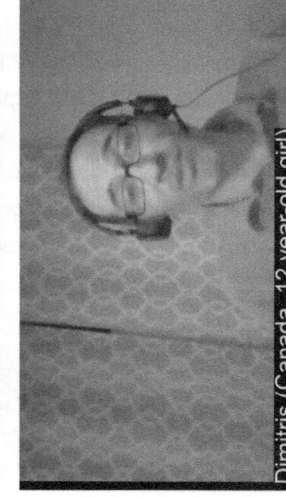

Dimitris (Canada, 12 year-old girl)

Video 2 Parents of children with KCNQ2-DEE (Kara Boulter, Dimitri Lazardis, Jenny Son, Claire Audibert, Mark Fitzpatrick) discuss family life with this neurological disorder.

A video transcript can be found in the Appendix. The video file is available at www.cambridge.org/weckhuysen-george

While the vast majority of patients experience seizures early in life, 32% of KCNQ2 Natural History survey respondents indicate their child is no longer experiencing seizures and does not require anti-seizure medications. Sixty-eight percent of patients require ongoing treatment with anti-seizure medications, which for many provides seizure freedom for months or even years. However, 12% have uncontrolled seizures, many beyond early childhood. As the community has gained increasing representation from older patients, the historically held clinical view that seizures in KCNQ2-DEE are self-limiting (which was based on experience with benign familial neonatal epilepsy) is clearly not true for many cases of KCNQ2-DEE.

> *My child still has seizures at least once a week, if not more. She's on epilepsy medications, which have helped but not stopped the seizures.*
>
> Mother of a 10-year-old girl in the United Kingdom

This type of outcome is not unusual among KCNQ2-DEE patients. Seizures take an enormous toll on families, who must remain vigilant. For example, the mother of a 7-year-old in Georgia reported that during the night, when her son's seizures occur, she and her husband must take turns watching him, and both developed anxiety and depression requiring treatment. This mother had to step back from a full-time position as a teacher to be a caregiver.

The other perspective gained with increased patient experience is that there is not a definite correlation between seizure activity and cognitive impairment. The mother of a 34-year-old patient in Poland noted that her daughter never had clinical seizures, yet her daughter was severely affected; whereas other individuals with recurrent seizures lasting years are among the higher functioning patients in the KCNQ2-DEE community.

Parents provided feedback about their children's gross motor skills. Many reported delayed or missed milestones as early signs of impairment. Of those participating in the KCNQ2 Natural History Study, 62% did not walk or, if under two years old, were experiencing moderate to severe delays. The experience of a mother of a two-and-a-half-year-old girl in Canada who "cannot hold her head up for more than a few seconds" is not unusual. For those who can walk, the interplay of cognitive limitations, including poor motor planning or limited receptive language, results in a mixed outcome.

> *My son has achieved a lot through repetition, especially activities he enjoys. He has learned to swim across the pool in a form of dog paddle, and can ski with guidance from a harness and tethers, but some simple acts like climbing into a car or stepping over an object in his way, remain a challenge.*
>
> Mother of 16-year-old boy in California, United States

Parents try various types of therapies to help their children improve their strength and gross motor function. Seventy-seven percent indicated that their child receives regular physical therapy. For many, the ultimate goal is learning to walk. For others, it is simply improving muscle tone to gain better head control. Various equipment is used by caregivers at home. Items such as a "tomato chair" for sitting support, a standing frame, braces, orthotics, and various homemade devices to stimulate movement for the nonambulatory are commonplace.

Perhaps due to the wide range of phenotypes, or perhaps due to the lack of data supporting any particular therapeutic intervention, families have pursued a variety of therapeutic approaches. A mother of a 3-year-old daughter in Thailand is among those who have children participating in Vojta therapy. Many parents have tried hippotherapy for their children. Most people with KCNQ2-DEE enjoy being in water, and many parents have used swimming to help their children.

The majority of those with KCNQ2-DEE require near constant assistance with activities of daily living (**Fig. 4**). According to the KCNQ2 Natural History Study, only 3% of individuals can use a toilet independently and only 2% can dress themselves. When it comes to mealtime, fewer than a quarter can use a spoon and fork and/or drink from a cup. In the area of hygiene, 15% responded that their child could wash and dry their hands, while only 7% could brush their teeth independently. Of children with KCNQ2-DEE, 13% demonstrate some academic skills, 18% demonstrate an ability to write or scribble with a crayon, and 22% are able to use a touchscreen device.

In the face of these challenges, parents celebrate milestones, like a mother in Texas whose 18-month-old daughter can hold her bottle to feed herself and the mother of a 7-year-old boy in the Netherlands whose son can eat small pieces of bread by himself.

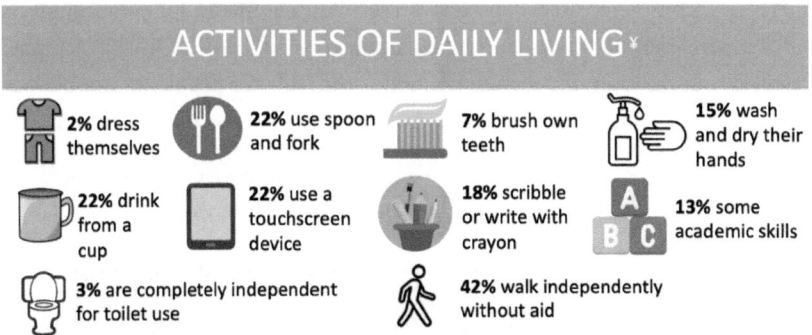

Figure 4 Summary of data related to activities of daily living from the KCNQ2 Natural History Study.

Those with KCNQ2-DEE continue to acquire knowledge and skills throughout their lives, although often, the gains come in bursts. The mother of a 10-year-old daughter in Colorado says the structure and intensity of Applied Behavioral Analysis (ABA) therapy proved invaluable. This mother also reported that the COVID-19 pandemic lockdown provided an unexpected opportunity, because she spent 30 hours per week in online school and therapy lessons with her daughter, who made significant academic gains. The child, who is nonverbal, can now identify all the letters of the alphabet visually and phonetically, is demonstrating pre-reading skills, and can also count from 1 to 20.

Some aspects of daily living activities may be more difficult. The mother of an 11-year-old Florida boy says her son can put on underwear and shorts by himself, but needs help with shirts, socks, shoes, and jackets.

> *My son is not able to grasp a utensil to eat his meals, but is able to use assistive technology to let us know when he wants more juice, or he is hungry, etc. He uses an eye gaze, voice output device that does not require physical assistance to navigate.*
> Mother of a 21-year-old man in Connecticut, United States

The KCNQ2 Natural History Study found that nearly 75% of families report their child has limited or no language, creating hardships for the patients and their families.

> *Nonverbal [and] only makes babbling sounds. Our main challenge is when he is in pain or sick or uncomfortable because he does not have any way of letting us know what is bothering him.*
> Mother of a 7-year-old boy in Georgia, United States

Some children with KCNQ2-DEE use augmentative speech devices, including Picture Exchange Communication (PEC) or smart-phone/tablet applications such as TouchChat. However, because of the global impact of the disease, alternative communication approaches are often hampered by poor cognition and limited fine motor skills. Parents often rely on their ability to decipher gestures, but this communication method is difficult for people at school or in the wider community.

> *My number one worry ... is definitely communication. She comprehends a lot of what we say, but she can't tell us what she's saying so she has major fits when we don't understand her.*
> Mother of a 3-year-old girl in the United States

Language matters and even a single word can have tremendous power. A 31-year-old English woman with KCNQ2-DEE can use 'pub' appropriately to convey her simple desire to spend time at the local pub.

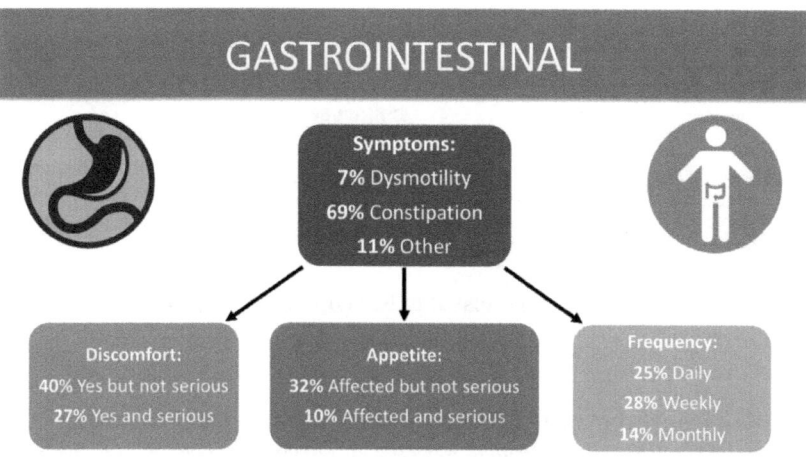

Figure 5 Summary of data related to gastrointestinal issues from the KCNQ2 Natural History Study.

Gastrointestinal (GI) issues are common among those with KCNQ2-DEE, according to families (**Fig. 5**), as described by Dr. Berg [7]. Risk factors include limited mobility, medications, and the ketogenic diet, although the main factor responsible for GI symptoms is not clear. Parents report that their children experience difficulty swallowing, excess drooling, reflux, constipation, and poor gut motility. Nearly 85% of the respondents to the KCNQ2 Cure Alliance survey say their child has constipation, which is often a daily concern. GI issues are reported across patients independent of age, mobility, muscle tone, or method of feeding (tube feeding, typical diet, or ketogenic diet). Parents report that GI issues cause their children considerable pain.

The mother of an adult daughter in the United Kingdom says her daughter has been on various medicines for "gut dysmotility" since she was eight months old. Her daughter was PEG-fed from the age of 9 to 18. Now 31 years old, her daughter's problems are so severe they have occasionally led to vomiting.

Some children with KCNQ2-DEE have remarkably sunny dispositions, according to their parents. But other families report that their children's challenging behaviors are one of the most difficult features of the disorder (**Fig. 6**). In the KCNQ2 Cure Alliance survey, 41 parents responded to questions about behavior. The behavioral difficulties vary widely, and are impacted by each individual's disposition and by their level of cognitive function. Patients with higher level functioning and greater awareness appear more frustrated, and possess the ability to display that frustration physically, unlike patients with more limited motor function or cognitive ability. Further complicating this picture, behavior can be inconsistent. Puberty can be an especially challenging period concerning behavior, but younger children with KCNQ2-DEE also struggle.

BEHAVIOR

Autism

17% Have features
20% Have a diagnosis

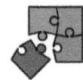

Difficult Behaviors

28% Frustration
8% Disobedience
8% Physical aggression
17% Temper tantrums
4% Verbal Aggression

21% Transition difficulties
19% Repetitive behaviors
35% Eyes-on supervision
15% Approach strangers
5% Not sharing

Figure 6 Summary of data related to behavioral issues from the KCNQ2 Natural History Study.

My child hits herself on the head. Usually very easily and for different reasons: attention, provocation, when she fails to do something, when something is forbidden to her.

Mother of a 3-year-old girl in Germany

My child hits/throws/bites/scratches when in meltdown. This happens when he is overwhelmed and has high anxiety. There is no reasoning with him when he is like this.

Mother of a 12-year-old boy in the United Kingdom

The mother of a 16-year-old girl in Australia diagnosed with ASD and KCNQ2-DEE, reported that her daughter was prescribed medicines for her self-injurious behaviors, which included banging her head against the wall. She later enrolled their daughter in intensive ABA therapy that has improved her behavior, academic ability, and demeanor.

Frustration can be expressed in other ways by those with limited mobility, such as hand biting. Vocalizing (yelling, screaming) can also be a feature of KCNQ2-DEE.

[My daughter is] very angry and upset when told "no." She goes through phases where she gets so upset about little things that she'll cry and scream at the top of her lungs but then is not able to calm herself back down which leads into usually 10–15 minute fits and sometimes longer, [but] overall her behavior is really good. She loves to hug and kiss anyone.

Mother of a 3-year-old in Missouri, United States

Sleep disturbances are common in KCNQ2-DEE (**Fig. 7**). Over half of those surveyed reported that their child awakens during the night at least three times per week, and some up to ten times a night. While seizures disrupt sleep in some cases, the majority suffer from unrelated sleep disturbances. With disrupted sleep and concerns about seizures, it is no surprise that the majority of parents indicated that they use some sort of electronic sleep monitor for their child.

SLEEP

Sleep disturbances
3 or more nights per week:
5% seizures
49% non-seizure awakenings
29% nocturnal restlessness

Monitoring child's sleep
63% monitor their child's sleep
23% co-sleep with child
55% audio or video monitor

Figure 7 Summary of data related to sleep issues from the KCNQ2 Natural History Study.

Concerns about sleep also appear to have a significant impact on caregivers. Parents may suffer from exhaustion, and may struggle to both work and parent after frequent nights of broken sleep.

Over half of parents surveyed by the KCNQ2 Natural History Study indicated that their child has two or more symptoms of autonomic nervous system dysfunction (**Fig. 8**). These include difficulty regulating temperature, sweating, respiration, salivating, and cardiac function. Approximately two-thirds of respondents to the survey report that their children drool or have excess saliva. A mother in Florida said, "*Getting people to understand her situation is tough because she looks like an average child until she starts drooling or acts differently.*"

When the KCNQ2 CURE Alliance survey asked parents to list the activities that their children enjoyed the most, music and water (swimming or bathing) were most common, consistent with the findings of the KCNQ2 Natural History Study (**Fig. 9**). Depending on their abilities, children enjoy anything from swimming to splashing in a bathtub. Musical interests include listening to songs, shaking shakers or bells, and singing for those who are verbal.

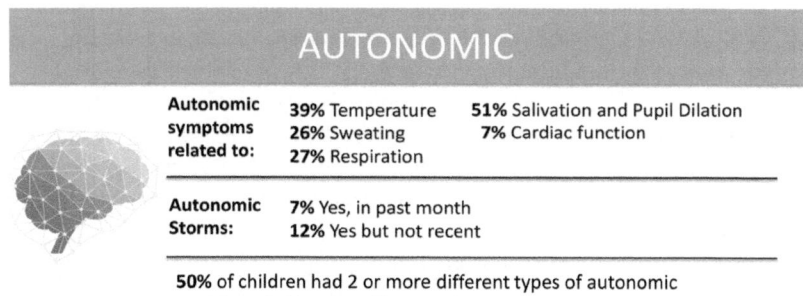

AUTONOMIC

Autonomic symptoms related to:	**39%** Temperature	**51%** Salivation and Pupil Dilation
	26% Sweating	**7%** Cardiac function
	27% Respiration	

| Autonomic Storms: | **7%** Yes, in past month |
| | **12%** Yes but not recent |

50% of children had 2 or more different types of autonomic symptoms in the preceding month.

Figure 8 Summary of data related to autonomic nervous system dysfunction from the KCNQ2 Natural History Study.

Positive Behaviors

39% Happy/Sweet/Affectionate
19% Showing concern
21% Get along with adults

Activities Enjoyed

81% Listening to music   27% Singing songs
71% Playing with water   23% Coloring
77% Being sung to   25% Playing an
60% Being read to   instrument

Figure 9 Summary of data related to positive behaviors and enjoyable activities from the KCNQ2 Natural History Study.

Vestibular stimulation also seems to be important for those with KCNQ2-DEE. About a third enjoy rocking back and forth, a number similar to those who like to ride in a car and those who like swinging on a swing. Many parents of children who are ambulatory volunteered that their children also like jumping on a trampoline. Regardless of their physical abilities, children with KCNQ2-DEE also are reported to enjoy bright lights, watching television and videos, getting tickled, and reading books.

Impact on Families

For parents, receiving a diagnosis of KCNQ2-DEE is akin to being hit with a meteor. Parents who were asked about the impact of KCNQ2-DEE on their family commonly use the word 'stress' in their answers, including enormous stress, financial stress, stress that they are not doing enough, and stress about health (**Fig. 10**). The impact of KCNQ2-DEE on the family is reflected in quotes from a variety of parents from around the world.

There is a 180-degree change in our way of life .... [W]e are most of the time sad and try to find happiness from little things.

Mother of a 5-year-old boy in Greece

It changed the type of house we live in, where we live, what type of neighborhood we could afford that was safest for our son.... It shapes family dynamics and our son's relationships with his grandparents. We don't travel for major family events like bar mitzvahs and weddings together. We are more isolated from our extended family than we might otherwise be. We don't vacation beyond a rare weekend ... and when we do, we need to stay on lower floors, and to know where the hospital is. His sister has learned to be a caregiver as a young teen. Our family is ok, we are strong, and close, but our son's diagnosis and related symptoms ... have had a profound impact on our family now and will into the indefinite future. We don't even have adequate savings and retirement tucked away yet and we are about 50 years old. My husband and I feel like it is a constant race against time.

Mother of an 11-year-old boy in Florida, United States

Having a child with KCNQ2 has profoundly affected our family, severely restricting our ability to spend time with friends, relatives, and to do anything that requires leaving home. It's extremely difficult to find qualified and competent caregivers to provide respite; [the] majority of our daughter's

FAMILY IMPACT

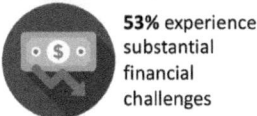 **53%** experience substantial financial challenges

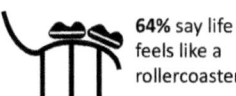 **64%** say life feels like a rollercoaster

 **60%** of parents experience moderate to severe fatigue

Figure 10 Summary of data related to impact on families from the KCNQ2 Natural History Study.

care falls on us (the parents), and often two people are needed to provide the care that she needs. Our days are tightly scheduled in accordance with medication and feeding schedule and her multiple other medical and sensory needs. This has placed a severe strain on our marriage and turned both myself and my husband into 24/7 caregivers for our daughter, without any hope for relief in the future. My biggest fear is that should my daughter outlive us, there will be no other caregivers capable of looking after her.
Mother of a 6-year-old girl in Canada

Parents will move mountains – even leave their state, territory, or country – to get the best care for their children. The mother of a 10-year-old Florida girl described the anguish of leaving Puerto Rico to get better medical care for her young daughter. The burden of caring for a child with KCNQ2-DEE without the help of family and a support system can pose additional hardships.

It's easy to think of the stress of having a teenager in diapers, the logistics and planning involved for taking simple family vacations, or even the difficulties of just a trip to the shopping center. We often opt to stay home for ease of managing, depending on the day and how she is coping with sensory details. We don't have external caregivers, so "getaways" are not a part of our daily lives. On the flip side, KCNQ2 has helped us all be more compassionate and consider what others might be facing, even if it's not apparent on the surface. We are all more patient and willing to help each other as a family. When one is struggling, the rest step up.
Mother of a 14-year-old daughter in Texas, United States

Initially it turned our world upside down but now it's just become the norm. Thankfully his seizures are under control and as long as he's happy we try to do everything we did before. Don't get me wrong, going places can be a challenge but we know what he needs and we just take more stuff than a typical family.
Mother of a 6-year-old boy in Arizona, United States

KCNQ2-DEE also affects families' work life. Juggling work and raising children is a tall order for any parent, but it can capsize families who have a child with KCNQ2-DEE. Many parents have had to quit work altogether, work fewer hours, or change the type of work they do, after having a child with KCNQ2-DEE.

> *KCNQ2 has really turned our lives upside down. ... I've had to leave work. So, we are only a one-income family.*
>> Mother of a 2-year-old boy in Australia

Parents who have more than one child also worry about the impact on siblings. The mother of a 5-year-old boy in Greece explained that her son's, *"older sister thinks that we care mostly for the KCNQ2 child."* An Australian mother of three whose youngest son has KCNQ2-DEE says her little boy's older siblings have witnessed seizures and the experience was traumatic. In contrast, there are cases in which there is a positive impact on siblings.

> *Our older daughter went into therapy as her career choice ... as an occupational therapist. Our older son is amazing with his little brother .... [Our son with KCNQ2] has young cousins that talk about seeing children in wheelchairs at their school and they talk to other kids in their class about kids that just have different needs but it doesn't make them different. He's had quite the impact on our family and all for the better.*
>> Mother of an adult child with KCNQ2-DEE in Arizona, United States

Concern for the future is expressed eloquently by one mother of a child with KCNQ2-DEE,

> *The stress of our son's unknowns health-wise impacted our lives first, it was quite a shock with a lot to learn to accept and adjust to; I had to completely change careers and sacrifice my earning potential (my husband did not and I think it's important to note that difference); our finances suffered and our life expectations and plans changed (like rarely taking a real family trip to learn/ vacation, buying a certain type of home near advanced medical resources, and making sure our son could get into a special school that could handle his needs appropriately). The stress is continuous and never lets up, because we can never really leave him unsupervised ever, even in our own home. The stress also relates to the future, because we worry about how we're going to take care of him when we're older and if we can find a safe group home for him to live in that will not be abusive and will meet his needs; that actually frightens us.*
>> Mother of a child with KCNQ2-DEE in Florida, United States

The KCNQ2 Cure Alliance is constantly amazed and inspired by the resilience of KCNQ2-DEE families, despite the overwhelming challenges that they and their children face every minute of each day. When parents and caregivers were asked about "silver linings," there were ample answers.

> *It is hard to think of an area of our family unaffected by KCNQ2. Every area of life became limited, but we eventually found ways to work beyond those limits. For example, we couldn't travel or get to very many places easily, so*

we got a small farm with animals, a garden, and lots of room to play so that we could have people come to us, even camp here so that we can 'vacation' with our family.

Mother of a 12-year-old girl in Washington, United States

She makes me realize the small things in life that can bring everyone happiness. I've become more empathetic since having a child with KCNQ2.... Every time she smiles or laughs, she brings us joy. When she hits a mini milestone, we get excited for her.

Mother of a 4-year-old girl in New Zealand

Basic Science of *KCNQ2* and *KCNQ3*

The original observations that led to the discovery of *KCNQ2* and *KCNQ3* as disease-causing genes encoding voltage-gated potassium (K_V) channel subunits responsible for neuronal M-current, is a fascinating multidisciplinary journey. In the next few paragraphs, the historical milestones that sculpted our current understanding of the pathophysiology of *KCNQ2*- and *KCNQ3*-related epilepsies are reviewed to highlight how research in distant and apparently unrelated scientific fields have converged to generate an astonishing series of seminal discoveries.

As recently reviewed [8], the dissection of the specific components responsible for the complex neuromodulatory effects exerted by the neurotransmitter acetylcholine drew considerable attention among neurophysiologists in the 1970s, mainly because of their enormous physiological relevance for central and peripheral nervous system function. In sympathetic neurons from rats [9] and frogs [10], acetylcholine released from preganglionic cells triggered muscarinic receptor-dependent slow excitatory post-synaptic potentials (sEPSPs), in addition to the well-studied fast nicotinic excitatory post-synaptic potentials (fEPSPs). These sEPSPs were accompanied by an apparent reduction in input resistance, suggestive of a fall in potassium ion (K^+) conductance, but also by a facilitation, or sometimes induction, of repetitive action potential firing. Because this K^+ conductance was suppressed by activation of M1, M3, or M5 subtypes of muscarinic receptors, it was named M-current. Activated M-current opposes cell depolarization by incoming stimuli, therefore inhibiting neuronal hyperexcitability and causing spike frequency adaptation during sustained depolarizations [11]. Muscarinic receptor activation, by suppressing M-current, depolarizes cell membranes and enhances membrane excitability, causing tonic neuronal firing. M-current accounts for a relatively minor fraction (<5%) of the total delayed rectifier K^+ current in neurons, and is not easy to record as it is heavily modulated by endogenous factors not easily reproducible under standard experimental conditions. Nonetheless, suppression of M-current can dramatically affect neuronal excitability because few other conductances are open at membrane voltages where M-current operates.

Following discovery of M-current in sympathetic neurons (**see Video 3**), similar currents were subsequently described in mammalian sensory neurons, as well as in central neurons such as hippocampal pyramidal neurons, olfactory cortex pyramidal neurons, and human neocortical neurons [8]. Moreover, similar currents were also demonstrated in gastric tissues, an observation that sparked investigations of M-current in smooth muscle cells [12].

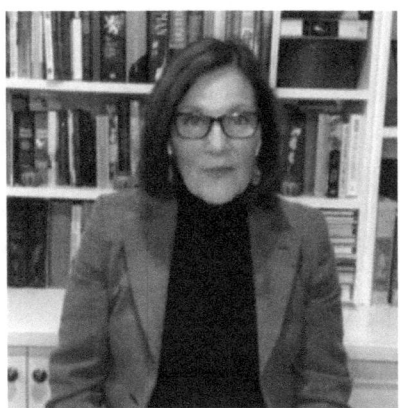 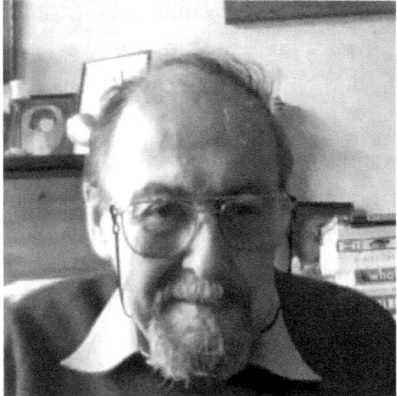

Sara James   David A. Brown, Ph.D.

Video 3 David A. Brown, Ph.D. (Professor Emeritus, University College London) discusses discovery of the M-current.

A video transcript can be found in the Appendix. The video file is available at www.cambridge.org/weckhuysen-george.

Despite its important function, the identification of the molecular components contributing to neuronal M-current (and to its diversity) was not easy, especially considering that voltage-gated K^+ channels exhibit the highest functional and molecular diversity among mammalian ion channels. Analogies between some functional properties of M-current and those of several other K_V channels (particularly those of the ether-a-go-go [eag] gene family) proved inconsistent, and the final answer had to wait for the solution to an issue arising in a completely different scientific field, namely the understanding of the genetic basis for a rare form of familial epilepsy, then called benign familial neonatal convulsions (or benign familial neonatal epilepsy), but recently reclassified as self-limited familial neonatal epilepsy (SLFNE) [13].

Self-limited familial neonatal epilepsy is an autosomal dominant genetic epilepsy syndrome characterized by seizure onset in the first week of life, focal sequential seizures (which remit spontaneously around five months of age), and normal neurodevelopmental outcome. Sporadic (nonfamilial) cases of the syndrome have also been described and likely have the same genetic etiology. The first family with SLFNE reported in 1964 had nine affected members who experienced their first seizures on the third day of life but then remitted spontaneously after a few weeks or months [14]. Between 1964 and 1989, around 30 families with SLFNE were reported, all showing autosomal dominant inheritance. The specific chromosomal abnormality in these families was identified in 1989, when linkage analysis enabled mapping of the gene in one of the largest families to the long arm of chromosome 20 (20q13.2) [15]. Linkage to this genetic locus was soon confirmed in several other families, and the SLFNE syndrome that maps to chromosome 20q was designated EBN1 (Epilepsy Benign Neonatal, type 1). In one of the few SLFNE families that did not link to chromosome 20, an additional locus on 8q24 was identified, and this syndrome was designated EBN2 [16]. Mapping of the chromosomal regions affected in EBN1 and EBN2 led to the identification of the specific gene defects by two groups simultaneously (one in Europe and one in the United States) in 1998. The genes involved were named *KCNQ2* [2,17] and *KCNQ3* [3] (see **Video 4**), respectively, because both had sequence homology to another gene, *KCNQ1*, which is associated with autosomal dominant (Romano-Ward syndrome) or recessive (Jervell and Lange-Nielsen syndrome) forms of congenital long QT syndrome [18]. Two additional members of the KCNQ gene subfamily were later characterized: *KCNQ4*, which is responsible for rare forms of autosomal dominant deafness [19], and *KCNQ5* [20], in which pathogenic variants have been recently found in rare sporadic cases of later-onset severe epilepsies [21].

KCNQ1-5 genes encode for K_V7 voltage-gated potassium channel subunits ($K_V7.1$-$K_V7.5$), which assemble as tetramers of identical (homotetramers) or compatible (heterotetramers) subunits similar to other K_V channels. Each K_V7 subunit has a topological arrangement with six transmembrane segments (S1–S6), with intracellular amino (N)- and carboxyl (C)-termini. The region encompassing

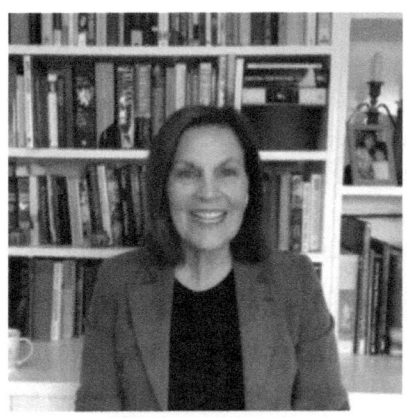
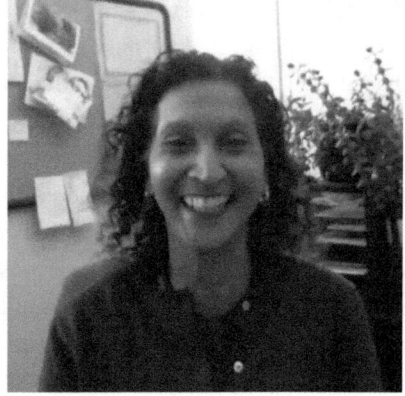

Sara James   Nanda Singh, Ph.D.

Video 4 Nanda Singh, Ph.D. (Laboratory Director, Myriad Genetics) discusses discovery of *KCNQ2* and *KCNQ3* genes in epilepsy.

A video transcript can be found in the Appendix. The video file is available at www.cambridge.org/weckhuysen-george

S1–S4 segments forms the voltage-sensing domain (VSD), while the S5–S6 segments and the intervening linker form the ion-selective pore (pore domain). As in other K_V channels, the S4 segments in K_V7 subunits contain from four to six positively charged arginine residues separated by two to three uncharged residues. However, unlike other K_V channels, the third arginine is replaced by a neutral glutamine residue. The K^+ selectivity filter in K_V7 channels has the canonical glycine-tyrosine-glycine (GYG) sequence. K_V7 channel function at various cellular sites and developmental stages is influenced by accessory subunits characterized by a single membrane-spanning domain and encoded by the *KCNE* gene family. Secondary structure analysis of the C-terminal region predicts four α-helices (A, B, C, and D), conserved in all K_V7 family members. Sites have been identified within the C-terminus that determine heteromeric and homomeric channel assembly, interaction with regulatory molecules (see section on Regulation of M-current and $K_V7.2/K_V7.3$ channels), subcellular localization, and binding of accessory proteins [20].

In parallel with the genetic discoveries of *KCNQ2* and *KCNQ3*, $K_V7.2$ and $K_V7.3$ subunits were heterologously expressed in *Xenopus* oocytes and in mammalian cells, and these experiments demonstrated functional heteromultimeric channels with distinct biophysical and pharmacological characteristics consistent with neuronal M-current [22]. Homomeric $K_V7.2$ channels carry robust K^+-selective currents activated by depolarization at membrane potentials around −50 mV, exhibit slow activation and deactivation kinetics, and lack significant inactivation. By contrast, currents carried by $K_V7.3$ homomers are small and activate at more negative potentials (−60 mV) [22,23]. At the single-channel level, $K_V7.3$ channels show the highest opening probability and unitary conductance among K_V7 members, a difference attributable to the different affinity of $K_V7.2$ and $K_V7.3$ subunits for the critical regulator phosphatidylinositol 4,5-bisphosphate (PIP_2, see section on Regulation of M-current and $K_V7.2/K_V7.3$ channels) [12]. Expression of $K_V7.2$ and $K_V7.3$ subunits in the same cell generates currents with amplitude approximately 10 times larger than that expected from the simple summation of the currents produced by the $K_V7.2$ or $K_V7.3$ homomers [22,23]. A higher opening probability of $K_V7.2/K_V7.3$ heteromers when compared to $K_V7.2$ homomers, together with a 2–3-fold increase in the number of channel-forming subunits expressed at the membrane, contributes to this potentiation.

Based on similarities in tissue expression pattern, biophysical properties, and pharmacological characteristics between native M-currents and those carried by the newly identified K_V7 subunits, it was concluded that, at least in adult sympathetic neurons, heteromeric assembly of $K_V7.2$ and $K_V7.3$ subunits represented the molecular correlate of the M-current [22]. SLFNE-causing variants in either KCNQ2 or KCNQ3 were found to decrease the currents carried by heterologously expressed channels incorporating $K_V7.2$ or $K_V7.3$ subunits [2,3,17], a result consistent with the "breaking" role of M-current on neuronal excitability. After more than 20 years of work, it is now clear that this assumption cannot be generalized to all neurons at each developmental stage. Several studies have converged on the idea that the molecular composition of functional K_V7 channels might not be necessarily fixed in the nervous system, but rather is dynamic and flexible across development, brain regions, cell types, and disease states, allowing some neurons to express $K_V7.2$ and $K_V7.3$ homomers [24,25]. Despite these refinements, it is undisputable that these early discoveries have set the groundwork for our current understanding of the molecular pathophysiology of M-current, paving the way for the further translational and clinical work, which is discussed in the next section.

Pharmacology of the M-current

Neuronal hyperexcitability is a common feature of different neuropsychiatric disorders such as epilepsy, neuropathic pain, amyotrophic lateral sclerosis, manic and anxiety states, attention deficit hyperactivity disorder, addiction to psychostimulants, depression, and many others. Therefore, pharmacological activation of M-current, a powerful means to suppress neuronal hyperexcitability, may represent an innovative treatment strategy in these diseases. On the other hand, compounds acting as M-current blockers, by increasing neuronal excitability and boosting the release of several neurotransmitters (including dopamine, serotonin, and glutamate) [26–28] may ameliorate the cognitive decline occurring in neurodegenerative diseases such as Alzheimer's disease, in which deficits in specific neurotransmitters is considered a major pathogenic event. The identification of compounds used both in vitro and in vivo as prototypic M-current activators or blockers largely preceded identification of the molecular target.

The first selective K_V7 blocker, linopirdine (DUP-996), was synthesized in the 1980s [29], in an attempt to provide "cognition enhancing" effects that could potentiate stimulus-evoked but not basal release of several neurotransmitters and increase the learning and memory performance of laboratory animals. Linopirdine was proposed to be potentially useful for the treatment of neurodegenerative conditions caused by neurotransmitter deficits such as Alzheimer's disease. However, clinical trials in Alzheimer's disease did not show efficacy [30], probably because of the suboptimal pharmacokinetic properties of the drug and its low potency in blocking M-current. DMP-543 and XE-991, two second-generation functional analogs of linopirdine, are more potent than linopirdine and are extensively used in research laboratories to reduce M-current in vitro and in vivo, although no clinical investigation in humans has been carried out with these drugs. Both linopirdine and XE-991 do not display selectivity among channels assembled from different K_V7 subunits, including the cardiac $K_V7.1$ subunit. Additional compounds with greater sub-type selectivity have recently been described, as recently reviewed [31].

Flupirtine was the first K_V7 activator [32,33]. This nonopioid, centrally acting analgesic has been clinically used in Europe since 1984 as an analgesic with muscle-relaxing properties. Because of rare cases of fatal liver injury, the Pharmacovigilance Risk Assessment Committee of the European Medicines Agency recommended to withdraw the marketing authorization of flupirtine-containing drugs in 2018. In addition to being effective in animal models of nociception, flupirtine exerted anticonvulsant effects against pentylenetetrazole (PTZ)-induced seizures. Furthermore, small-scale uncontrolled clinical trials suggested that flupirtine was effective in reducing seizure frequency in patients resistant to conventional anticonvulsants. However, anticonvulsant effects occurred at doses ten times higher than those producing analgesia [34]. To separate the analgesic from the anticonvulsant activity, flupirtine derivatives were synthesized and evaluated for their anticonvulsant activity. The most potent derivative was retigabine (renamed ezogabine in the United States), which exhibited anticonvulsant activity in a broad spectrum of seizure models, including PTZ-induced seizures, maximal electroshock, audiogenic seizures in DBA/2J mice, and seizures produced by amygdala kindling [34]. Such broad spectrum of anticonvulsant activity in experimental animals distinguished reti-gabine from other anticonvulsants available at the time, suggesting a novel mechanism of action. The first observation that retigabine modulated voltage-gated K^+ channels was published in 1997 [35], although the specific class of K^+ channel targeted by the drug was unknown. The cloning of *KCNQ* genes revealed the molecular targets for retigabine [12,31].

The main effects of retigabine on K_V7 channels are a hyperpolarizing shift of the voltage-dependence of channel activation, slowing of deactivation, acceler-ation of activation, and an increase in maximal current density. Retigabine-induced effects on the voltage-sensitivity of K_V7 currents appear to be of variable amplitude in channels formed by different K_V7 subunits, being greatest for $K_V7.3$, intermediate for $K_V7.2$, and least for $K_V7.4$ homomeric channels [31]. Importantly, retigabine does not affect $K_V7.1$. This high degree of subunit selectivity is attributed to retigabine binding in a hydrophobic pocket located between the cytoplasmic parts of the S5 and the S6 transmembrane domains in the open channel configuration. Within this cavity, a lipophilic interaction is established between the fluorophenyl ring of retigabine and the aromatic side chain of a tryptophan present at the intracellular end of the S5 helix (W236 in the $K_V7.2$ sequence). In $K_V7.1$, this tryptophan is naturally substituted by the smaller and less hydrophobic leucine, thus explaining their retigabine insensitivity and the cardiac safety of this compound [31].

The potency of retigabine for activating $K_V7.2/K_V7.3$ channels ($EC_{50} \sim 1–3$ µM) is compatible with the free drug concentration range achieved in plasma during standard treatment. Based on its unique anticonvulsant profile in experimental animals and mechanism of action, the antiepileptic efficacy of retigabine has been evaluated in numerous human studies, leading to its approval for clinical use in 2011 (trade name Trobalt in Europe or Potiga [ezogabine] in the United States) as adjunctive treatment of focal-onset seizures in patients who respond inadequately to alternative treatments. However, despite a favorable benefit–risk profile acknowledged by the European Medicines Agency in 2016, the manufacturing company (GlaxoSmithKline) discontinued the commercialization of retigabine after June 2017 mostly because of its limited usage.

Several drawbacks are likely responsible for the limited clinical success of retigabine. Activation of $K_V7.4$ and $K_V7.5$ channels expressed in genitourinary smooth muscle cells was the plausible explanation for urinary retention, a frequently reported side effect. Retigabine has a short half-life in plasma and is metabolized by phase II enzymes (by acetylation and N-glucuronidation) with little involvement of the cytochrome P450 system. Consequently, retigabine requires three-times-a-day dosing. The drug has poor brain penetration because of its limited lipophilicity, and relatively high drug doses are required. A major clinical concern with retigabine is its tendency to cause retinal and muco-cutaneous blue-gray discoloration [36]. Although the mechanism for this toxic effect remains poorly understood, one hypothesis is that UV radiation may cause photodegradation and oxidation of the aniline ring, which may lead to the formation of colored deposits in skin and eyes [37]. Despite these limitations, treatment with retigabine has been suggested as a form of targeted therapy in severe forms of *KCNQ2*-related epilepsies, and a randomized, double-blind, placebo-controlled trial has recently been initiated with a pediatric formulation of the drug.[2]

In the last decade, several research groups have developed retigabine analogues with improved physico-chemical, pharmacokinetic, or pharmacodynamic properties, as well as K_V7 activators originating from pharmacophoric structures distinct from retigabine and there are recent reviews on these topics [31,38,39].

---

[2] ClinicalTrials.gov Identifier: NCT04639310.

Regulation of M-current and $K_V7.2/K_V7.3$ channels

In addition to muscarine-sensitive cholinergic receptors, many neurotransmitters and neuromodulators suppress the M-current, including substance P, angiotensin II, ATP, glutamate, and serotonin [40]. In fact, a common feature that emerged from the studies in the 1980s and 1990s was that neuromodulation of the M-current is a widespread phenomenon that is not simply restricted to sympathetic neurons but is present in almost all neurons that express an M-current, and that most neurotransmitters and neuromodulators act through Gq/11 protein-coupled receptors [40]. Activation of Gq/11 protein-coupled receptors leads to the activation of phospholipase C (PLC) and downstream activation of inositol 1,4,5-trisphosphate (IP3) and diacylglycerol (DAG) followed by protein kinase C (PKC) (**Fig. 11**) [40]. As a result, for many years, most investigators focused their attention on the role of PKC, IP3, and cytosolic Ca^{2+} as M-current modulators. This led to apparently conflicting data, as the M-current was sensitive to PKC blockers or activators in some neurons but not others. The mystery was resolved a few years after the molecular identification of the M-current. A series of papers in early 2000 showed that the polyanionic phospholipid PIP_2 controls the activity of $K_V7.2$ and $K_V7.3$, and the M-current [40].

The PIP_2 hydrolysis by PLC gives rise to inositol trisphosphate (IP3) and diacylglycerol (DAG). Thus, any Gq/11 protein-coupled receptor upon IP3 and DAG activation would lead to depletion of PIP_2 in the plasma membrane. This initial depletion could lead to the inhibition of $K_V7.2$ and $K_V7.3$, providing an explanation for the convergence of M-current inhibition by a plethora of neurotransmitters and neuromodulators. The identification of PIP_2 as a key signaling molecule also led to the recognition that PIP_2 is required for the gating of the M-current and K_V7 channels in general. Consequently, K_V7 channels should be considered voltage gated and PIP_2 activated, with PIP_2 being an allosteric activator. $K_V7.2$ channels in particular are very sensitive to PIP_2 plasma membrane levels, as their affinity is almost ten-fold lower than that of $K_V7.3$ channels. As a result, the sensitivity of the M-current for PIP_2 depends on its subunit composition, with $K_V7.2$ homomers having low affinity, $K_V7.3$ the highest, and $K_V7.2/K_V7.3$ heteromers somewhere in between. Although it is not fully clear what distinguishes $K_V7.2$ and $K_V7.3$ affinity, significant efforts have identified PIP_2 binding sites at the S2–S3 linker, S4–S5 linker, proximal part of S6, and A–B helix linker found in the C-terminus. Additionally, the contribution of the different PIP_2 binding sites appears to shift as the channel opens and closes, allowing different PIP_2 sites to stabilize distinct $K_V7.2$ conformations [20,41].

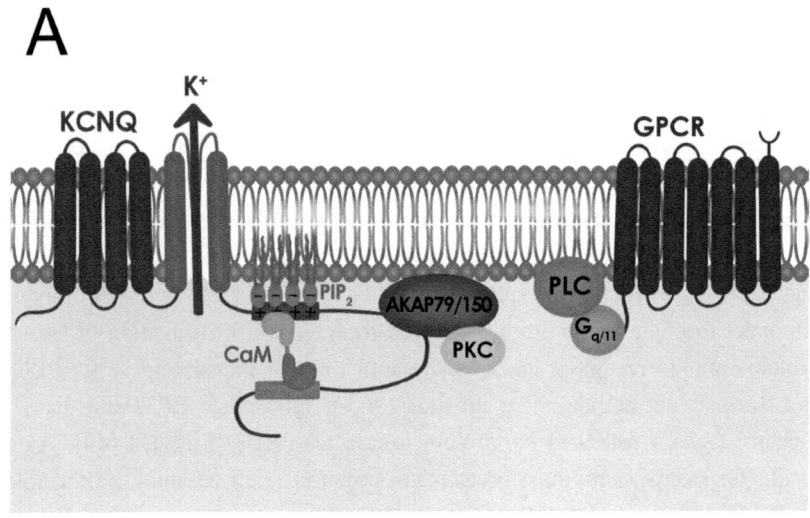

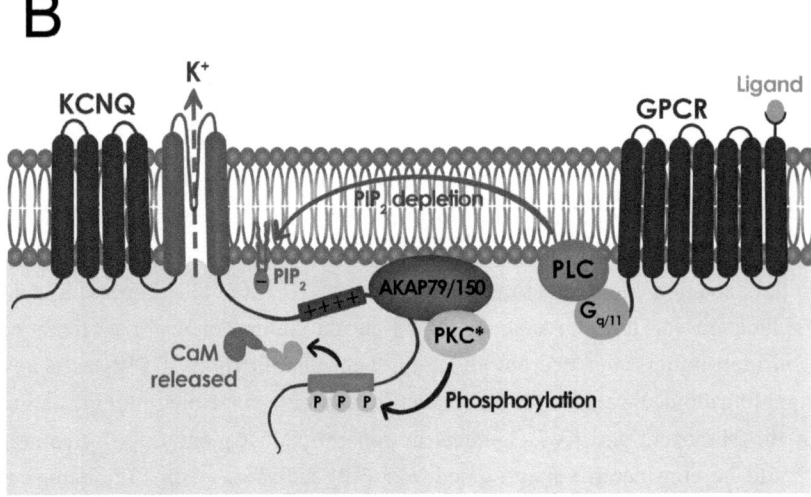

Figure 11 Signal transduction mechanisms controlling M-current activity. (A) M-current activity (KCNQ channel) when G-protein coupled receptor (GPCR) is inactive. (B) M-current activity is suppressed when GPCR is active.

The distribution of PIP$_2$ binding sites, typically positively charged lysine and arginine residues, also explains the multiple functions of PIP$_2$ in regulating K$_V$7.2 channel properties. For instance, PIP$_2$ depletion primarily affects the probability of K$_V$7.2 channel opening, consistent with PIP$_2$ sites found in S6 and the C-terminus. Similarly, high levels of membrane PIP$_2$ increase the maximum open probability of K$_V$7.2 channels, and shift its voltage-activation toward more negative membrane potentials, as expected for PIP_2 binding in the S4–S5 linker and distal S4 that may enhance coupling between the pore domain and the voltage sensor [42]. Another feature of the PIP_2 binding sites is that they overlap with or are in close proximity to known phosphorylation sites (i.e., PKC), binding sites for A-kinase-anchoring protein (AKAP), and cal- modulin [20]. As a result, the affinity of K_V7 channels for PIP_2 is tunable and dynamic. Indeed, Hoshi and colleagues demonstrated that PKC activation leads to the phosphorylation of serine-534 and serine-541. Replacement of these serine residues with alanine prevents phosphorylation by PKC and blunts the ability of muscarinic G protein-coupled receptors to inhibit the M-current and $K_V7.2$ [20,43].

Understanding the synergy between PIP_2, PKC, and calmodulin provides important background to explain how PKC controls the muscarinic modulation of $K_V7.2$. Several studies demonstrated that calmodulin can act as an auxiliary subunit for ion channels, and $K_V7.2$ channels bind calmodulin [20,43]. Calmodulin regulates multiple facets of $K_V7.2$ channel function including trafficking, orchestrating tetramerization with $K_V7.3$ channels, and controlling the affinity of $K_V7.2$ for PIP_2. Calmodulin binds to the A and B helix of the C-terminus and can undergo a conformational change upon Ca^{2+} binding. Consequently, phosphorylation of serine-541 by PKC weakens the interaction of calmodulin with $K_V7.2$, dislodging calmodulin from the channel (**Fig. 11**) [43]. The loss of calmodulin lowers the affinity of $K_V7.2$ for PIP_2. Therefore, activation of muscarinic receptors impacts $K_V7.2$ channels directly by rapidly depleting PIP_2 (a consequence of activating PLC) and indirectly by activating PKC phosphorylation of $K_V7.2$, which reduces channel affinity for PIP_2 by dislodging calmodulin. This dual regulation explains why $K_V7.2$ channels are particularly sensitive to muscarinic activation, or neuromodulation by other Gq coupled receptors (**Fig. 11**). The significance of this interaction is further highlighted by studies using knock-in mice in which serine-559 in mouse $K_V7.2$ is replaced by an alanine. These mice are less sensitive to muscarinic receptor-induced seizures and exhibit memory deficits [44].

PIP_2, calmodulin, and PKC are not the only regulators of $K_V7.2$ channels. Protein kinase A (PKA) has also been implicated in the control of $K_V7.2$ channel properties [45]. A canonical PKA phosphorylation site is located in the $K_V7.2$ N-terminus (serine-52). Presently, the regulation of the M-current by PKA is unclear, as the M-current is not regulated by PKA in most neurons. However, this lack of modulation might be cell-type specific or due to the fact that some $K_V7.2$ channels are tonically phosphorylated by PKA. In addition to PKA, arginine methylation can also regulate $K_V7.2$ channel activity. This post- translational modification has received little attention over the years, but recent work has shown that multiple C-terminus arginine residues can be methylated, reducing their positive charge and, in turn, their ability to interact with PIP_2 in the inner leaflet of the plasma membrane [46]. Lastly, activation of oxidation of cysteine residues in the S2–S3 linker may enhance K_V7 channel activity, raising the possibility that $K_V7.2$ activity could be bidirectionally regulated [47]. Further work is needed to determine the extent to which *KCNQ2* variants alter the interactions of $K_V7.2$ with modulatory partners and whether disease-associated variants alter the responses of $K_V7.2$ to different neuromodulators.

Although much of the field's focus has been to identify the mechanisms that regulate M-current activity, earlier work demonstrated that M-current modulation also regulates the release of monoamine neurotransmitters such as norepinephrine and dopamine, in addition to glutamate and gamma-aminobutyric acid (GABA) [26,27]. Thus, $K_V7.2$ loss-of-function variants increase excitability not only by changing intrinsic neuronal properties, but also by increasing the levels of neuromodulators in the brain.

Physiological function of $K_V7.2$ channels in neurons

$K_V7.2$ channels are expressed throughout the central, peripheral, and enteric nervous systems. With very few exceptions, $K_V7.2$ channels are found in all neuronal cell types, independent of whether they are excitatory, inhibitory, glutamatergic, GABAergic, glycinergic, or monoaminergic. The widespread distribution of $K_V7.2$ channels was clearly demonstrated by two complementary studies, one from Rudy and colleagues using in situ hybridization and another by Cooper and colleagues using immunohistochemistry [48,49]. Both groups reported expression of $K_V7.2$ channels throughout the forebrain, thalamus, caudate putamen, and brainstem. Follow-up studies have also shown expression of $K_V7.2$ channels in the spinal cord as well as in sensory neurons innervating various organs including the lung, bladder, and gastrointestinal tract (**Fig. 12**) [20].

Further work by multiple groups also established that $K_V7.2$ channels have a unique somatoaxonal distribution [20,43]. In particular, $K_V7.2$ channels are highly enriched at the axon initial segment (AIS), a site of high sodium channel expression and where action potentials are generated. In unmyelinated axons, $K_V7.2$ channels are found across the axon, whereas in myelinated axons $K_V7.2$ channels are highly expressed in the nodes of Ranvier. $K_V7.2$ has an ankyrin-binding domain at the C-terminus, and ankyrin G is highly expressed in axons (**Fig. 12**). Although $K_V7.2$ channels should be considered axonal, this does not preclude additional localization in dendrites or soma. For instance, some reports have suggested that $K_V7.2$ channels are present in the spines of layer 2/3

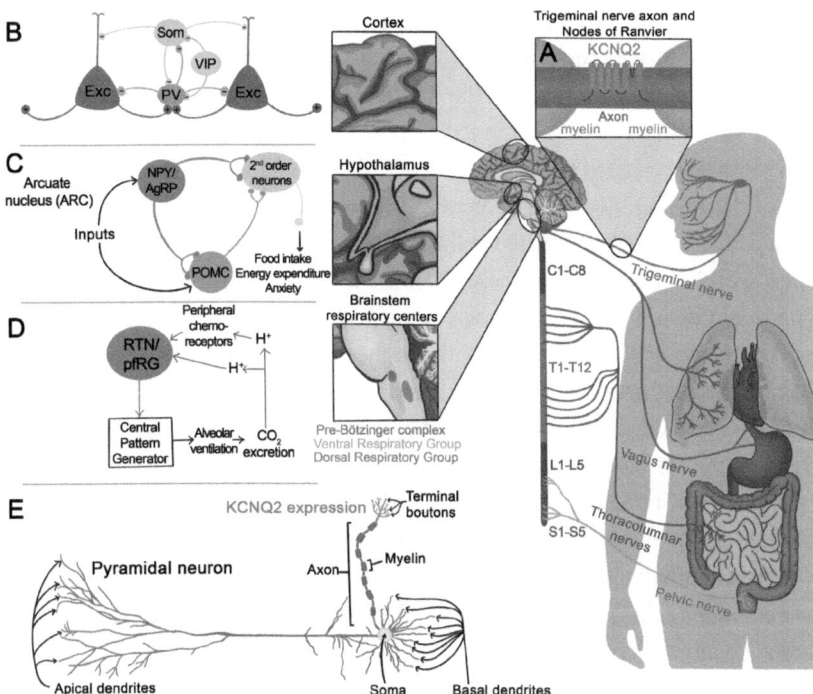

Figure 12 Summary of KCNQ2 channel anatomic and subcellular localization.

pyramidal neurons [50]. However, the current consensus is that $K_V7.2$, as well as $K_V7.3$, follow a somatoaxonal distribution, with axons having an almost ten-fold higher concentration of $K_V7.2$ [51].

The function of $K_V7.2$ channels in neurons underlies two primary K^+ driven processes, the M-current and the medium afterhyperpolarization (mAHP) [11]. Pharmacological [52,53] and genetic [54,55] evidence indicate that the mAHP, which typically activates following an action potential or a burst of multiple action potentials, depends on $K_V7.2$ and $K_V7.3$ channels. To fully understand the role of $K_V7.2$ channels in neurons and how *KCNQ2* pathogenic variants might alter neuronal physiology, we must consider the dual role of $K_V7.2$ channels.

M-current – As discussed, M-current is a slow-activating and non-inactivating K^+ conductance, which activates before neurons reach the threshold for action potential firing. As a result, M-current is considered to act as a brake on neuronal activity. $K_V7.2$ channels concentrate primarily in axons. Indeed, electrophysiological recordings from layer V pyramidal neurons demonstrated that K_V7 channels are the dominant K^+ conductance in axons at subthreshold membrane potentials [56]. Thus, $K_V7.2$ channels can contribute to neuronal excitability in three ways.

First, $K_V7.2$ channels contribute directly to setting the resting membrane potential of the AIS. Blocking K_V7 channels with XE991 caused an approximately 5–6 mV depolarization in the AIS, and this effect was not observed when XE991 was applied to the soma [51,56]. Second, M-current affects the availability of voltage-gated sodium channels at the AIS indirectly through modulation of the resting membrane potential. Because a substantial fraction of AIS sodium channels are inactivated at the resting potential, activation of M-current will lower the proportion of these channels available to fire action potentials. This would be reflected as a change to the peak action potential amplitude and the rise of the action potential, as the higher the sodium channel density the faster the rate of action potential activation. Changes in sodium channel availability would also alter the speed of action potential propagation down the axon [51]. Lastly, M-current limits the influence of the persistent subthreshold sodium current to neuronal excitability [57]. Most neurons exhibit a persistent subthreshold sodium current that acts to promote neuronal excitability and pacemaker activity. A key function of M-current, and therefore $K_V7.2$ channels, is to counteract the influence of the subthreshold persistent sodium current and dampen neuronal excitability.

Medium afterhyperpolarization (mAHP) – As discussed earlier, the mAHP becomes activated after a neuron has fired a burst of activity (a few action potentials) or in neurons that have a pronounced afterdepolarization (e.g., CA1 and layer V pyramidal neurons). The primary function of the mAHP is to prevent runaway neuronal firing [11]. Consequently, robust activation of the mAHP induces spike frequency adaptation, which is characterized by a decrease in the firing frequency during sustained depolarization. Depending on the size of the mAHP, the adaptation could lead to neuronal silencing. Thus, any changes in the mAHP could alter the firing behavior of a neuron.

We can understand the dual role of $K_V7.2$ channels in neuronal physiology by considering the $K_V7.2$ channel gating properties in general. Neuronal $K_V7.2$ channels activate slowly in comparison to an action potential (tens of milliseconds rather than a few milliseconds), allowing for a very small fraction of $K_V7.2$ channels to contribute to the repolarization phase of an action potential. However, neurons with a prominent afterdepolarization can stay depolarized for tens of milliseconds, allowing $K_V7.2$ channels to activate. Indeed, blocking $K_V7.2$ channels pharmacologically or ablating them genetically leads to a prolonged afterdepolarization. A longer-lasting afterdepolarization allows neurons to fire another round of action potentials, thus increasing their excitability.

Although slow activation kinetics prevent $K_V7.2$ channels from activating during the repolarization of the action potential, they are ideally suited to preventing subthreshold depolarization. This, along with their lack of inactivation, allows

$K_V7.2$ channels to act as a powerful brake on incoming activity and decrease the rate of subthreshold depolarization. This is particularly important early in development when neurons have a much more depolarized membrane potential. Such a membrane potential would probably lead to pronounced inactivation of A-type and D-type K^+ currents, currents that typically control neuronal firing properties.

The dual role of $K_V7.2$ channels in neuronal excitability also becomes important when attempting to interpret the impact of *KCNQ2* pathogenic variants on neuronal excitability. For instance, variants that decrease surface expression or the probability of opening would decrease both the subthreshold M-current and the mAHP. However, variants that shift the voltage-activation of $K_V7.2$ channels to more depolarized membrane potentials might decrease the activity of only the M-current, leaving the mAHP intact [58]. In summary, predictions regarding the effects of *KCNQ2* variants must consider both the M-current and the mAHP, recognizing that not all variants would alter their properties similarly.

$K_V7.2$ Function in Different Circuits in the Nervous System

$K_V7.2$ channels are expressed throughout the nervous system and in multiple cell types. Some of the major findings on $K_V7.2$ channels pertaining to different neural circuits are described here.

A series of studies soon after the discovery of *KCNQ2* determined the localization of $K_V7.2$ channels in the brain. Early on, researchers recognized that $K_V7.2$ channels are not restricted to one cell type; rather, they are expressed by multiple cells including glutamatergic, GABAergic, and monoaminergic neurons [49]. Consistent with their widespread expression, K_V7 channel inhibitors or activators either increase or dampen the activity of pyramidal neurons as well as somatostatin-positive and vasoactive intestinal peptide-positive interneurons in the forebrain [59,60]. Importantly, genetic deletion of *Kcnq2* in mouse pyramidal neurons and parvalbumin-positive interneurons increased their firing rates [55,61]. Such *Kcnq2* deletions led to a higher frequency of spontaneous excitatory and inhibitory events, consistent with $K_V7.2$ regulation of axonal excitability. In addition to the use of *Kcnq2* knock-out mice, studies have used mice expressing loss-of-function *Kcnq2* variants. For instance, Peters et al. (2005) used a mouse line expressing a dominant-negative pore variant (G269S) to demonstrate that $K_V7.2$ channels are responsible for both the M-current and the mAHP [54]. Additional studies using human *KCNQ2* variants or knock-in mice further confirmed that $K_V7.2$ dysfunction leads to increased forebrain pyramidal neuron activity and enhanced network excitability that could manifest in learning and memory deficits [62–64].

Another theme emerging from the aforementioned mouse studies is that the effects of $K_V7.2$ channels in neuronal excitability do not persist throughout development. For instance, Peters et al. (2005) found that conditional expression of a *Kcnq2* loss-of-function pore variant (G269S) in mice leads to early lethality and hyperexcitability when the variant is expressed prior to birth or within the first few of weeks of life [54]. However, expression of the same pore variant after the second of week of life led to mice that survive to adulthood, albeit with some behavioral deficits [65]. These two studies raised the possibility that *KCNQ2* loss of function might have strong effects early in development, setting a cascade of events that lead to compensation and remodeling of the forebrain networks later in life. Indeed, a recent study using neurons derived from human induced pluripotent stem cells (iPSC) found substantial transcriptome changes leading to upregulation of K^+ channels, presumably to counterbalance the hyperexcitability phenotype due to decreased $K_V7.2$ channel activity [66]. Thus, the effects of $K_V7.2$ channel dysfunction in forebrain neurons and networks might change over time, becoming less severe as the network matures.

An emergent concept about $K_V7.2$ and $K_V7.3$ channels is that their levels are dynamic and change depending on the behavioral state of the organism. This has been demonstrated in the hypothalamus, a brain region critical for sleep, stress, and importantly, energy homeostasis. A key circuit that controls energy balance is the central melanocortin system that includes the arcuate nucleus neuropeptide Y/agouti gene-related protein (NPY/AgRP) neurons as well as pro-opiomelanocortin (POMC) neurons (**Fig. 12**) [67]. The arcuate nucleus is proximal to the third ventricle and median eminence having access to circulating hormones (insulin, leptin) important for energy homeostasis. As NPY/AgRP and POMC neurons have receptors for these circulating hormones, they act as first-order neurons. A series of studies have shown that stimulation of NPY/AgRP neurons leads to food-seeking behaviors, whereas activation of POMC neurons decreases food intake [67]. Activation of NPY/AgRP also leads to additional behavioral effects, most notably reduction in anxiety [68]. The majority of NPY/AgRP neurons express $K_V7.2$ and $K_V7.3$ channels and exhibit M-current [69]. Importantly, previous studies have shown that fasting, which leads to increased firing activity of NPY/AgRP neurons, is associated with lower $K_V7.2$ and $K_V7.3$ expression and lower M-current [69]. Indeed, several of the effects of fasting on NPY/AgRP neuron excitability are recapitulated by blocking $K_V7.2/K_V7.3$ channels or by knocking down *Kcnq3* [69,70]. Similar to NPY/AgRP neurons, corticotrophin-releasing hormone (CRH) neurons found in the paraventricular nucleus of the hypothalamus increase their activity depending on the behavioral state of the animal, in this case, following stress. CRH neurons are part of the hypothalamic–pituitary–adrenal axis; thus an increase in their activity results in elevated levels of circulating glucocorticoid hormones. The increase in CRH neuron activity following stress was partly due to downregulation of the M-current and $K_V7.3$ levels [71]. Thus, depending on the behavioral state of the animal, $K_V7.2$ and $K_V7.3$ levels change allowing neurons to tune their firing properties. This also suggests that *KCNQ2* pathogenic variants are likely to alter the properties of hypothalamic neurons that in turn might dysregulate homeostatic control of energy balance, stress, and sleep.

Developmental and epileptic encephalopathy associated with $K_V7.2$ has been attributed primarily to loss-of-function variants [24,72]. However, recurrent pathogenic *KCNQ2* variants (R201C) that stabilize the activated state of the channel to produce a gain-of-function effect have also been identified [73]. Patients with the R201C variant display severe myoclonus and early profound hypoventilation due to reduced chemoreflex, followed by multifocal seizures, impaired development, and early mortality. Apnea has also been reported in patients with *KCNQ2* loss-of-function, although with less severity than in gain-of-function variants. The mechanism responsible for abnormal respiration associated with *KCNQ2* gain-of-function variants may affect the brainstem circuits involved in the control of breathing.

Key components of the respiratory control circuit are located in the medullary portion of the brainstem. Respiratory rhythm is generated by premotor neurons in the pre-Bötzinger complex that control inspiration and a subset of neurons located in the parafacial respiratory group that regulate active expiration [74]. The output of neurons that regulate inspiration and expiration is relayed to respiratory motor neurons to influence the rate and depth of breathing. Central chemoreceptors located in several regions, including the nucleus of the solitary tract, medullary raphe, and retrotrapezoid nucleus (RTN), and peripheral chemoreceptors located in the carotid bodies regulate respiratory rhythm based on changes in CO_2/H^+ and O_2 levels (**Fig. 12**). $K_V7.2$ channels are found within the respiratory control centers, and therefore, $K_V7.2$ dysfunction might alter some or all of the circuits associated with breathing regulation. Currently, the greatest knowledge about the $K_V7.2$ channels and breathing stems from work in the RTN, a key region for sensing changes in CO_2/H^+ [74].

RTN neurons are intrinsically chemosensitive, increasing their firing activity in response to changes in CO_2 and, consequently, pH [74]. Although $K_V7.2$ channels are pH sensitive, their pH sensitivity is outside the range for chemoreception. $K_V7.2$ channels control the basal firing frequency of RTN neurons, in part by dampening the activity of the TRPM4 channel, a Na^+ and K^+ permeable channel that controls the oscillation frequency of RTN neurons [75]. Thus, a gain-of-function *KCNQ2* variant might hyperpolarize the membrane, making it more difficult for neurons to respond to changes in extracellular pH.

Phenotypes, Variant Hotspots and Disease Pathophysiology

In the 20 years following their discovery, insights into $K_V7.2$ and $K_V7.3$ function in humans have been provided by the convergence of molecular genetics and of detailed phenotyping of large cohorts with various types of epilepsy and neurodevelopmental disorders. Given that $K_V7.2$ and $K_V7.3$ form heterotetramers, one might hypothesize similar effects from variants in the *KCNQ2* and *KCNQ3* genes, but differences have been observed between the two genes' profiles.

Pathogenic variants in *KCNQ2* and *KCNQ3* lead to an array of diseases characterized by epilepsy and/or neurodevelopmental disability with variable severity. Remarkably, the phenotypic spectra are paralleled by the genotype and, in the case of missense variants, by the functional properties of the variant channels. The different conditions caused by pathogenic variants in *KCNQ2* and *KCNQ3* can be considered along two phenotypic spectra associated with opposing functional mechanisms: (1) impaired potassium channel function (LoF), and (2) enhanced potassium channel function (GoF) (**Fig. 13**). Moreover, the severity of the phenotype appears correlated with the degree of channel dysfunction. Importantly, however, it is clear that, in addition to spectra of severity within each condition, there is a range of outcomes even for identical genotypes, making prognostication challenging.

In general, pathogenic alterations in *KCNQ2* are more frequent and more severe than paralogous variants in *KCNQ3*. In a recent prospective cohort study in Scotland, *KCNQ2* was by far the most common single-gene neonatal-onset

Phenotypes by Genetic Mechanism

	Neonatal-Onset Developmental & Epileptic Encephalopathy	Self-Limited Familial Neonatal Epilepsy	Intellectual Disability Autism Spectrum Disorder Epilepsy	Neonatal Encephalopathy with Non-Epileptic Myoclonus; Infantile Spasms
KCNQ2	Dominant Negative Missense (*De Novo*)	Protein-Truncating Variants, or Loss-of-Function Missense (Dominantly Inherited)	Gain-of-Function Missense (*De Novo*)	Gain-of-Function Missense (*De Novo*)
KCNQ3	Biallelic Protein-Truncating, or Biallelic Missense (Recessively Inherited)	Dominant Negative Missense (Dominantly Inherited)	Gain-of-Function Missense (*De Novo*)	

Figure 13 Phenotypes associated with *KCNQ2* and *KCNQ3* pathogenic variants and the typical genetic mechanism. Variant classes and functional consequences are given for each gene in each phenotypic grouping, with typical inheritance provided in parentheses. The most severe phenotypes associated with certain gain-of-function missense variants in *KCNQ2* have not been reported in association with *KCNQ3*. Likewise, neonatal-onset DEE has only rarely been reported in association with biallelic *KCNQ3* variants.

epilepsy, with an estimated incidence of 1 per 17,000 live births [76]. Several potential mechanisms may explain the lower incidence of epilepsy-associated variants described for *KCNQ3* when compared to *KCNQ2,* and for the more severe clinical consequences associated with *KCNQ2* variants when compared to corresponding variants in *KCNQ3.* These include the different temporal pattern of expression of the two genes in the developing human brain, with *KCNQ2* being expressed earlier during fetal development than *KCNQ3.* Other factors such as epistatic compensation [72] may also account for differences in the reported numbers of variants. More importantly, these data reinforce the concept that *KCNQ2* and *KCNQ3* are not always expressed together in all neurons and at each developmental stage.

Functional Consequences of $K_V7.2$ and $K_V7.3$ Pathogenic Variants

Functional studies are of paramount importance to assess the potential pathogenicity of sequence variants, to reveal pathophysiological mechanisms of disease, and to investigate potential genotype-phenotype correlations. When studied in vitro, most *KCNQ2* and *KCNQ3* variants responsible for SLFNE and nonfamilial SLNE cause channel loss-of-function (LoF) [77]. The molecular mechanisms responsible for LoF are heterogeneous, and include reduced K^+ permeation when the variant affects residues located in the pore domain; lower open probability and faster closing kinetics for variants affecting critical gating residues in the voltage-sensing domain; changes in the affinity and/or functional regulation of the channel by cytoplasmic regulators such as syntaxin-1A, calmodulin, PIP_2, and others; mRNA instability by nonsense-mediated RNA decay or channel protein instability; and altered subcellular distribution such as when the interaction with axon-targeting signals or interacting proteins is disrupted. Nevertheless, irrespective of the mechanism evoked by each variant, haploinsufficiency, corresponding to M-current reduction of only 25% not compensated by the wild-type allele, has been postulated as the mechanism by which inherited variants in *KCNQ2* or *KCNQ3* lead to SL(F)NE [72]. By contrast, missense pathogenic *KCNQ2* variants associated with DEE exhibit more severe functional defects on channel function, suggesting that a dominant-negative effect could be responsible for more severe epilepsy phenotypes [78,79]. Subunits carrying these missense variants would decrease channel function more than 25%, because incorporation of even a single mutant subunit would "poison" the function of the entire tetrameric channel. Thus, together with additional genetic and epigenetic factors, the extent of mutation-induced derangement of $K_V7.2/ K_V7.3$ channel function appears as an important predictor of disease severity.

While SLFNE-causing pathogenic variants in *KCNQ2* appear to be randomly distributed throughout the gene, those causing DEE appear to be concentrated in four hotspots that represent channel domains exerting critical functional roles [41,80,81] including the S4 helix of the voltage-sensing domain (VSD), the pore domain containing the ion selectivity filter, the A-helix in the proximal C-terminus that binds PIP_2 and calmodulin, and the more distal B-helix of the C-terminus that provides an additional attachment site for calmodulin.

In addition to the LoF mechanisms previously described for both KCNQ2-SLFNE and KCNQ2-DEE, heterozygous de novo missense variants that cause gain-of-function (GoF) effects on channel activity have also been identified in severely affected patients with KCNQ2-DEE. These include R201C/H, R144Q, and R198Q. The R201C/H variants affect the second positively charged residue (designated R2) within the S4 segment of the voltage-sensing domain. Electrophysiological studies in heterologous cells revealed that channels formed by Kv7.2 subunits with these variants display larger peak current density than wild-type channels, a marked hyperpolarizing shift in the voltage-dependence of activation, and an acceleration of activation kinetics, collectively suggestive of an increased sensitivity of channel opening to voltage. Qualitatively similar, although quantitatively milder, functional effects have been described for R144Q located in the S2 segment (72) and R198Q, corresponding to the first arginine residue (R1) in the S4 segment [82]. These results further expand the emerging genotype–phenotype correlations between clinical severity and the extent of GoF demonstrated in vitro, given that milder/ intermediate phenotypes appear associated to less dramatic GoF changes (R144Q, R198Q), and more severe phenotypes are instead associated with the strongest GoF effects (R201C/H).

Reinforcing the distinct functional and pathophysiological role between *KCNQ2* and *KCNQ3* is the recent observation that de novo missense mutations located at the two outermost arginine residues in the voltage-sensor, of the $K_V7.3$ S4 segment (R227 and R230; corresponding to R198 and R201 in $K_V7.2$) occur in children presenting with global developmental delay, autism spectrum disorder (ASD), and frequent sleep-activated multifocal epileptiform discharges. When expressed in vitro, mutations at the R230 position in $K_V7.3$ (R230C/H/W) exhibit strong GoF effects, whereas qualitatively similar but milder effects were exhibited by R227Q, thus showing functional characteristics rather similar to those displayed by the corresponding variants in $K_V7.2$ subunits [73]. These results, consistent with the high degree of sequence similarity between $K_V7.2$ and $K_V7.3$ in the affected region, suggest an identical molecular mechanism responsible for the GoF effect in both subunits. However, it seems remarkable that, despite similar functional consequences of variants at positions R1 or R2 observed in $K_V7.2$ and $K_V7.3$, the clinical picture of patients carrying variants at these positions differs by gene, again pointing toward distinct functional roles exerted by these two K_V7 subunits during human neurodevelopment.

Enhanced neuronal excitability associated with $K_V7.2$ GoF variants seems paradoxical and has been difficult to explain and is a focus of research for many groups (**Video 5**). GoF variants in $K_V7.2$ may cause hyperexcitability by altering network interactions rather than intrinsic cell properties [83], and, in close similarity with other channelopathies such as the Dravet syndrome caused by mutation in *SCN1A* voltage-gated sodium channels, KCNQ2-DEE caused by

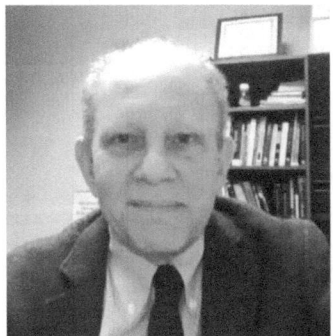
Edward Cooper, M.D., Ph.D.

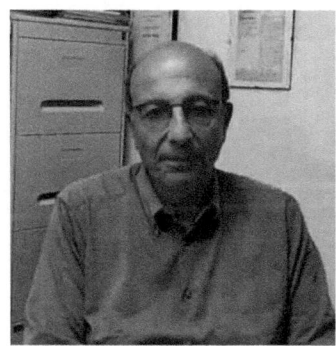
Maurizio Taglialatela, M.D., Ph.D.

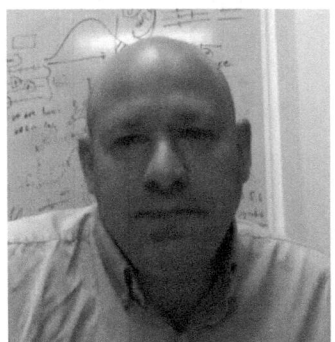
Anastasios Tzingounis, Ph.D.

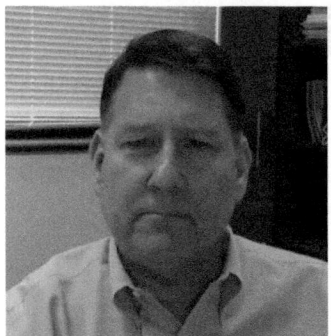
Alfred L. George, Jr., M.D.

Video 5 Panel discussion among researchers who study KCNQ2 biology (Edward C. Cooper, M.D., Ph.D., Baylor College of Medicine; Maurizio Taglialatela, M.D., Ph.D., University of Naples Federico II; Anastasios Tzingounis, Ph.D., University of Connecticut; Alfred L. George, Jr., M.D., Northwestern University).

A video transcript can be found in the Appendix. The video file is available at www.cambridge.org/weckhuysen-george

specific GoF variants might be regarded as an "interneuronopathy." Additional mechanisms to explain enhanced neuronal excitability caused by GoF mutations have been proposed including the activation of a recurrent neuron–astrocyte–neuron excitatory loop, faster action potential repolarization and sodium channel repriming, and overactivation of the hyperpolarization-activated nonselective cation current resulting in secondary depolarizations [84].

Genotype–Phenotype Correlations

Neonatal-Onset Epilepsy and DEE: *KCNQ2* and *KCNQ3* LoF-Associated Phenotypes

Neonatal epilepsy is the hallmark of disease caused by pathogenic variants in *KCNQ2* and *KCNQ3* that result in LoF. There are two main conditions. Certain dominantly inherited variants in *KCNQ2* and *KCNQ3* cause SLFNE, usually associated with good outcomes (e.g., resolution of epilepsy, normal development). At the other end of the spectrum, certain de novo missense and indel variants in *KCNQ2* are responsible for KCNQ2-DEE. While these two conditions are distinguished by stark differences in neurodevelopmental outcomes and epilepsy severity, the electroclinical features of the seizures are remarkably similar [85]. Moreover, clinically and electrographically, these features are distinct from the focal seizures typically observed in acute provoked seizures in neonates (**Fig. 14a**) [86].

In both KCNQ2-SLFNE and KCNQ2-DEE, seizure semiology is asymmetric tonic (or sequentially tonic then clonic), lasting 1–2 minutes (**Fig. 14b; Video 6 and Video 7**). The laterality varies among seizures, sometimes left and sometimes right, in the same patient. Perioral cyanosis caused by apnea during the seizures is typical. Ictal EEG shows diffuse attenuation with rapid spread of fast activity and pronounced post-ictal suppression [86], a pattern that is detectable by conventional EEG and amplitude-integrated EEG as well [88]. Seizures have a clinical component at presentation, and electroclinical dissociation (transition to subclinical seizures following treatment) is rare [86].

Seizures in neonatal-onset epilepsies associated with LoF variants in *KCNQ2* or *KCNQ3* tend to be poorly responsive to phenobarbital, levetiracetam, and benzodiazepines, treatments commonly used to treat seizures in the nursery. Instead, seizures respond best to sodium channel blockers, such as CBZ (also fosphenytoin, but maintaining adequate levels in infants may be challenging) [86,87,89]. Because seizures are commonly frequent at presentation, affected newborns are at risk for aggressive treatment protocols with repeated loads of anti-seizure medications and/or continuous infusions resulting in prolonged hospitalization if seizures are not controlled. Treatment with a sodium channel blocker, such as CBZ, is therefore recommended at the earliest clinical suspicion (**Fig. 14c**). Treatment is discussed further in later sections.

Self-Limited Familial Neonatal Epilepsy

Dominantly inherited neonatal epilepsy associated with good outcomes (SLFNE) was first described by Rett and Teubel in 1964 [14]. For many years

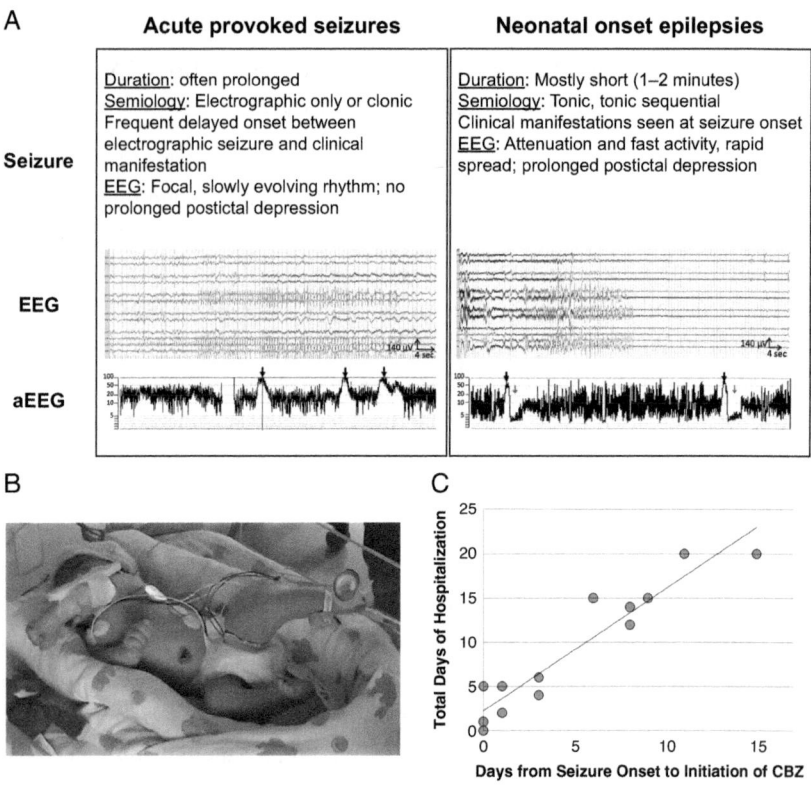

Figure 14 Electroclinical features of seizures in neonatal onset epilepsy and DEE caused by impaired function of *KCNQ2* or *KCNQ3*. (A) Summary of the clinical and electroencephalographic (EEG) features in acute provoked seizures and neonatal onset epilepsies. Black arrows indicate seizures; grey arrows indicate postictal depression. EEGs: gain, 10 µV/mm; high-frequency filter, 70 Hz; paper speed, 15 mm/s. aEEG, amplitude-integrated EEG. (B) Clinical semiology of seizures in neonatal-onset epilepsy resulting from impaired function of *KCNQ2* or *KCNQ3*: Asymmetric tonic posturing with apnea and desaturation that may subsequently evolve to asynchronous bilateral clonic movements. This is a newborn with SFNE caused by an inherited stop-gain variant in *KCNQ2* (c.807 G>A; p.Trp269Ter). (C) Length of hospitalization by time to carbamazepine (CBZ). In patients treated with CBZ in the neonatal period, the length of hospitalization was directly correlated with when CBZ was initiated, p < 0.01. Modified with permission from Cornet et al., 2021 (A) [86] and from Sands et al., 2016 (B, C) [87].

this epilepsy was called benign familial neonatal convulsions/seizures/epilepsy. To avoid giving the incorrect impression that seizures are ever benign, "self-limited" has been proposed in place of "benign." In this context, "self-limited" is meant to reflect the fact that seizures resolve after infancy. The name remains imprecise, however, as many individuals go on to have additional seizures later in life. Moreover, while the responsible pathogenic variants are usually inherited, mutations can arise de novo. Finally, some individuals can first present outside of the neonatal period. *KCNQ2* pathogenic variants have also been found in families with self-limited familial infantile epilepsy (SLFIE), in which seizures start around six months of age, and self-limited familial neonatal-infantile epilepsy (SLFNIE), in which seizures display an intermediate age of onset between the neonatal and the infantile periods [76]. Therefore, despite the name, it is important to recognize that the seizures in SLFNE may recur later in life, may not be inherited, and do not always start in the neonatal period.

In 1998, SLFNE was mapped to *KCNQ2* at 20q13.33 and *KCNQ3* at 8q24.22, and pathogenic variants were found that resulted in moderate impairment in potassium channel function in vitro [2,3,17,45]. SLFNE is associated with a variety of heterozygous frameshift, stop-gain, intragenic and whole-gene deletions, splice variants, and missense variants distributed throughout the *KCNQ2* gene. Notably, heterozygous truncating/deletion variants account for a substantial proportion (39%) of *KCNQ2* variants associated with SLFNE.[3] Less commonly, SLFNE is caused by heterozygous missense variants in *KCNQ3* (15 with good evidence, affecting 12 clustered residues) [90]. Heterozygous truncating *KCNQ3* variants have not been associated with a human phenotype. *KCNQ2* variants are responsible for the majority of SLFNE families (~ 80%), while inherited pathogenic *KCNQ3* variants are comparatively rare, accounting for approximately 5% of families [87,91]. Furthermore, de novo pathogenic heterozygous variants in *KCNQ2* have also been detected in sporadic cases of SL(F)NE, thus confirming a shared molecular etiology for both familial and nonfamilial cases. To date, SLFNE caused by these two genes cannot be distinguished from one another phenotypically.

Seizures in SLFNE are focal motor seizures characterized by asymmetric tonic semiology, sometimes evolving to clonic jerking (**Fig. 14a,b; Video 6**). Apnea accompanying tonic stiffening often leads to oxygen desaturation. The seizures last one to two minutes and begin during the first week of life. Whereas acute provoked seizures in neonates and seizures in KCNQ2-DEE typically start within the first 24 hours of life, seizure onset in SLFNE is most common at days two to four [86,92]. This hallmark delay in onset is quaintly captured by the historical term "fifth-day fits." An implication of this delay is that babies with SLFNE may present in the well-baby nursery or, in some cases, after discharge to home.

---

[3] www.rikee.org.

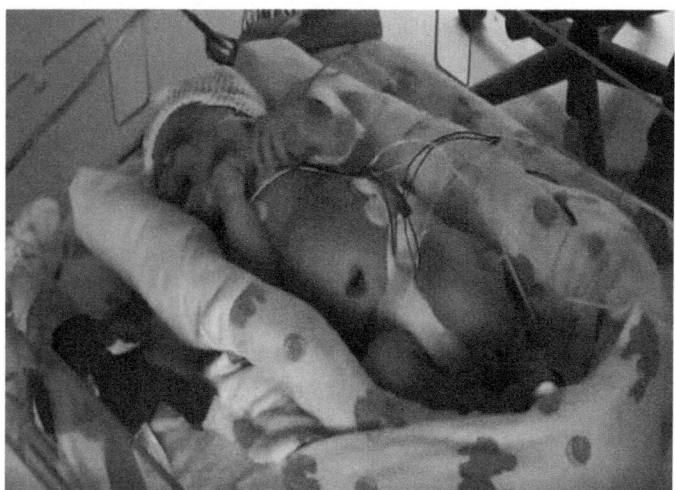

Video 6 Seizure in a newborn with SLFNE associated with a truncating *KCNQ2* variant (c.807 G>A; p.Trp269X). Semiology is tonic sequential. The baby initially extends the left upper extremity and then assumes a "sign of four" asymmetric tonic posture before onset of asynchronous bilateral clonic jerking. Cyanosis can be appreciated. Modified with permission from Sands et al., 2016 [87].
The video file is available at www.cambridge.org/weckhuysen-george

Family history, while obviously helpful, may not be immediately available, known or even present. Unless told about their history, parents may be unaware that they had seizures as newborns. Often, seizures and epilepsy are not openly discussed due to stigma. Neonates with seizures may be sent some distance to tertiary care centers and parents may not be immediately available. Penetrance of the condition is approximately 80%, so parents of affected newborns may not have had seizures themselves or may be unaware of their extended family history, particularly if the condition exhibits incomplete penetrance ("skips a generation") [91]. Finally, de novo founder mutations can occur, as for any gene, leading to noninherited variants and sporadic disease.

KCNQ2-associated seizures can be frequent, especially during the first days of life, and seizures every three to six hours is common, and higher rates have been observed [91,92]. The affected newborns are typically otherwise well in between seizures and have normal neurological exams, but this can change with the effects of sedating medications (e.g., phenobarbital loads). Brain imaging is likewise normal in SLFNE, in contrast to KCNQ2-DEE. The interictal EEG in the immediate aftermath of a seizure is abnormal but progressively improves, evolving from post-ictal suppression and then excessive discontinuity to near normal until disrupted by the next seizure.

Babies with SLFNE represented 2% of newborns with seizures in a cohort drawn from seven intensive-care nurseries in the United States [93]. As discussed, distinguishing these children from acute provoked seizures has important management implications, as inadequate control can lead to hundreds of seizures for 13% of cases [91]. Importantly, the distinctive seizure type can lead to a presumptive diagnosis and effective treatment with a sodium channel blocker prior to the return of genetic test results [86,87].

Seizures resolve for many infants by 6 months of age, but they may continue through the first 12–15 months of life [87,91,92]. In one study, seizure recurrence after infancy was originally estimated to occur in 10–15% of cases [92], but may be as high as 31% of individuals. Recurrent seizures may be triggered by fever in subsequent years, or present as epilepsy later in childhood or even in adulthood [91]. The rate of seizure recurrence later in life was greater in individuals with a higher burden of seizures in the neonatal period [91]. About 5% of reported families include affected members with epilepsy onset in infancy outside of the neonatal period [91,94].

Developmental outcomes are usually good overall for SLFNE, though it may be hard to predict at the time of presentation whether a child's course will be self-limited epilepsy or DEE. Some missense *KCNQ2* or *KCNQ3* variants in SLFNE families have more variable outcomes [95–100]. Missense variants in *KCNQ2* are also responsible for DEE, and outcomes in SLFNE may be best thought of as a spectrum that overlaps the milder end of DEE.

KCNQ2 Developmental and Epileptic Encephalopathy

KCNQ2-DEE is a neonatal-onset epilepsy that is almost always sporadic and is associated with a spectrum of neurodevelopmental disability, usually moderate to severe [101,102]. KCNQ2-DEE is the most common cause of neonatal epilepsy with encephalopathy, accounting for over 34% of cases that underwent genetic testing in a multicenter cohort, and about one-third of DEE cases with burst suppression on EEG [93,103]. It presents with seizures, hypotonia, and impaired visual attention in the very first days of life. The interictal EEG is abnormal, marked by excessive sharp waves and discontinuity exacerbated by seizures and sedating anti-seizure medications. Some cases have presented with seizures and EEG findings suggesting or even consistent with Ohtahara syndrome [103]. Indeed, shortly after the description of KCNQ2-DEE [101], other studies [104,105] reported the condition as Ohtahara syndrome. However, distinct from Ohtahara syndrome, neonates with KCNQ2-DEE do not have

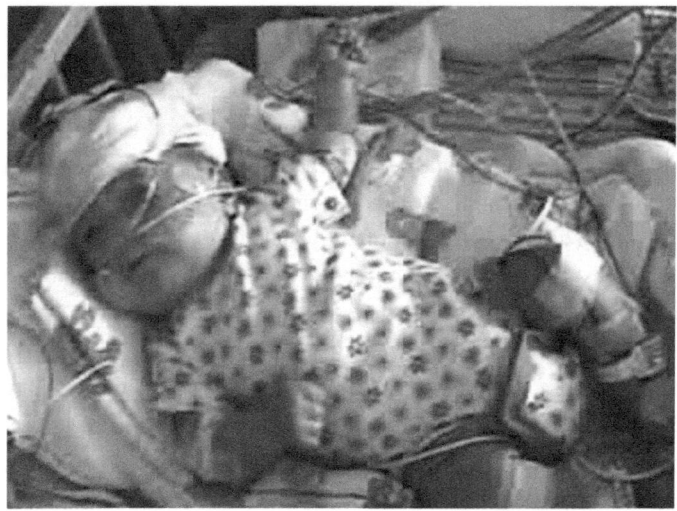

Video 7 Seizure in a child with KCNQ2-DEE associated with a missense *KCNQ2* variant (c.1734 G>C; p.Met578Ile). Seizure starts with left eye and head tonic deviation accompanied by left arm tonic contraction and chewing; this is followed by rightward head, eye, and buccal tonic deviation and arm and leg contraction. With permission from Numis et al., 2014 [85].
The video file is available at www.cambridge.org/weckhuysen-george

epileptic spasms. Instead, seizures are focal tonic and often accompanied by apnea and blood oxygen desaturation [85,89]. The seizures in KCNQ2-DEE are often clinically and electrographically similar to those of SLFNE: focal motor seizures characterized by asymmetric tonic posturing accompanied by apnea and sometimes progressing to clonic jerking evolving over one to two minutes (**Video 7**) [85].

Seizures often start within the first 24 hours of life placing infants with KCNQ2-DEE at risk of being mistaken for hypoxic-ischemic encephalopathy. Brain magnetic resonance imaging (MRI) may show T2 hyperintensities in deep nuclear structures (e.g., basal ganglia, thalamus) that later resolve, but does not show evidence of infarction and/or parenchymal hemorrhage indicative of acute symptomatic etiologies [102]. Interpretation by someone skilled in reading neonatal imaging studies is essential.

The typical electroclinical pattern of KCNQ2-DEE (**Fig. 14a**) can allow for early recognition prior to genetic test results [86]. This is important because seizures are frequent and response to most treatments is poor, potentially leading to prolonged hospitalizations. While there is interest in targeted treatment with the potassium channel activator ezogabine/reti-gabine [80], sodium channel blockers, such as CBZ, are currently the most effective treatment available for seizures and may allow for earlier dis-charge [86,89].

KCNQ2-DEE and SLFNE share seizure semiology, ictal EEG, and response to sodium channel blockers, but can be distinguished by the presence or absence of encephalopathy and by the interictal EEG and sometimes MRI findings with KCNQ2-DEE, as noted earlier. The situation may be difficult to interpret if the exam and EEG are obtained after use of sedating anti-seizure medications, such as phenobarbital, or in the setting of continuous infusions. Family history, if present, and the genotype, when it becomes available, can inform prognosis (**Fig. 13**). Some variant types may help predict outcome; heterozygous *KCNQ2* truncating variants and *KCNQ3* missense variants are typically associated with SLFNE. The clinical course associated with de novo missense *KCNQ2* variants is more challenging to predict, as they typically result in KCNQ2-DEE but can also cause SLFNE [106].

The spectrum of developmental outcomes in KCNQ2-DEE ranges from mild intellectual disability to profound neurodevelopmental disability (nonverbal, nonambulatory, without purposeful use of limbs, gastrostomy-tube dependent), with most reported cases falling in the moderate to severe end of the spectrum [101,102]. In a report of individuals surviving to adulthood, approximately 75% were nonverbal or had very limited speech, and about half were unable to walk independently [107]. The seizures tend to improve over the first two decades, becoming less frequent and more manageable than during the first months and years of life [107].

KCNQ2-DEE is a developmental and epileptic encephalopathy, which emphasizes the direct impact of the genetic variant on brain function in addition to the impact of seizures on the developing brain. It is not known to what extent early improved seizure control might affect developmental outcomes. One study found only weak evidence to support improvement in outcomes related to seizure control when correlating the duration of seizure freedom with dis-ability [6]. However, the impact of seizure burden during the peak incidence in the first months of life was not evaluated. Such studies are inherently challenged by the difficulty of controlling for genotype.

KCNQ2-DEE is most often caused by de novo missense and indel (in-frame deletion) variants in four hotspot functional domains (the S4 transmembrane segment, the pore, and the A-helix and B-helix in the C-terminus) [81]. These variants may act through a "dominant negative" mechanism [79] and exert a more profound impairment on channels in comparison to KCNQ2-SLFNE missense variants [78]. Predicting the pathogenicity and potential functional consequences of variants in *KCNQ2* can be aided by variant databases such as gnomAD,[4] the Rational Intervention for KCNQ2/3 Epileptic Encephalopathy (RIKEE) database,[5] and published reports detailing the effects of specific variants on hyperexcitability [66]. Despite these resources, prognosis for de novo KCNQ2 missense variants remains complex. Some benign variants may be novel and therefore not represented in databases. For most known pathogenic variants, few patients have been described (often not in detail and/or without long-term follow up). Moreover, even for recurrent variants, there is a spectrum of outcomes [106]. Thus, prognostic information should appropriately capture what is known, while also acknowledging what is not known.

KCNQ3 Developmental and Epileptic Encephalopathy

While heterozygous truncating variants in *KCNQ3* have not been clearly linked to a disease phenotype, neonatal-onset epilepsy and developmental delay has been reported with homozygous *KCNQ3* frameshift variants [108,109]; for example, a child with homozygous variants resulting in KCNQ3 F534Ifs*15. She was able to walk independently just before three years of age, but was not speaking in complete sentences by eight years and moderate intellectual disability was reported [108]. Neonatal onset epilepsy with a wide range of developmental severity was reported across three affected siblings with homozygous *KCNQ3* variants resulting in a frameshift (S407Ffs*27) [109]. The determinants of phenotypic variability in such closely related individuals are unknown. In another example of biallelic *KCNQ3* disease, early-onset epilepsy with severe nonverbal cognitive impairment and spastic quadriparesis has been reported in the setting of compound heterozygous for *KCNQ3* variants (V359L and D542 N) that impair PIP_2-dependent current regulation [110].

Overall, very few individuals with biallelic pathogenic variants in *KCNQ3* have been reported to date, but early impressions support a spectrum of neonatal onset developmental and epileptic encephalopathy with parallels to KCNQ2-DEE. Notably, contrary to *KCNQ3*, no homozygous truncating *KCNQ2* variants have been described in humans, probably indicating that absence of *KCNQ2* is not compatible with life.

KCNQ2 and *KCNQ3* GoF-Associated Phenotypes

A spectrum of complex neurodevelopmental phenotypes is associated with specific de novo heterozygous missense *KCNQ2* and *KCNQ3* variants that are considered GOF leading to channel activation at less-depolarized potentials

---

[4] https://gnomad.broadinstitute.org/.   [5] https://www.rikee.org/.

[82,83,111]. These disorders are characterized by developmental delay and variably severe impairments in cognition, language, and fine and gross motor function that come to clinical attention in the first two years of life. Some children may be diagnosed with autism spectrum disorder. Most individuals have an epileptiform EEG during childhood and some have seizures. Interestingly, and unlike the LoF-associated phenotypes, seizures are not universally present and do not occur in the neonatal period.

Neonatal Encephalopathy with Non-epileptic Myoclonus and Central Hypoventilation

The most severe of this group of disorders presents with a type of neonatal encephalopathy without seizures, characterized by non-epileptic myoclonus and a burst-suppression EEG pattern (**Fig. 15**) [73]. The condition is associated with variants that neutralize the second arginine residue in the S4 transmembrane segment of *KCNQ2* (R201C, R201H). There is the suggestion of a milder phenotype for R201H compared to R201C, but the number of patients reported is limited.

Neonates are encephalopathic and hypotonic with hyperreflexia and exaggerated startle. Paroxysmal attacks, consisting of massive reflex myoclonus triggered by tactile or acoustic stimuli and persisting beyond the duration of the stimulation, can be mistaken for seizure but are without an electrographic correlate [73]. Taken together, neonatal encephalopathy with a burst-suppressed EEG pattern and myoclonus might suggest the syndrome of early myoclonic encephalopathy (EME), but the massive, triggered, and persistent high-amplitude non-epileptic myoclonic jerking differs from the fragmentary, segmental, or erratic epileptic myoclonus that predominates in EME. The exaggerated startle is reminiscent of hyperekplexia, but in that condition there is no encephalopathy and EEG is normal.

Central hypoventilation and periodic breathing with apneic episodes along with risk for aspiration pneumonia are often associated with respiratory compromise, with the need for respiratory support and gastrostomy tube placement. These respiratory symptoms place the babies at risk for early death. Some patients were reported to develop diabetes insipidus in the first two months. Some had a cleft palate. MRI of the brain shows a thin corpus callosum, progressive volume loss and hypomyelination. One reported patient had subependymal heterotopias.

Neurodevelopmental impairment is profound. The EEG usually evolves from burst-suppressed to a high-amplitude disorganized background with multifocal epileptiform discharges (**Fig. 15b**) and most children develop infantile spasms. Response to standard treatments is poor with only partial response suggested for

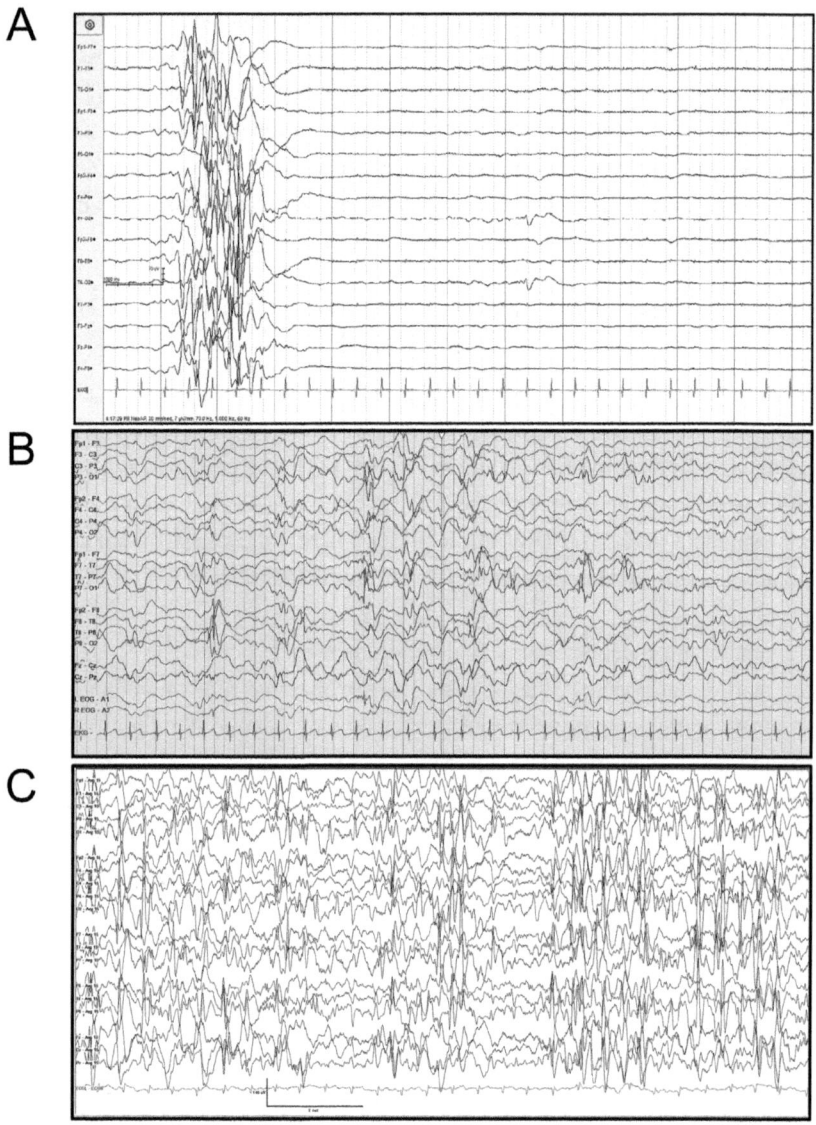

Figure 15 Electroencephalography (EEG) associated with gain-of-function (GoF) variants in *KCNQ2* and *KCNQ3*. (A) EEG (7 μV/mm) of a 2-day-old newborn with a GoF variant in *KCNQ2* (c.601C>T, p.R201C), showing a burst-suppression pattern. With permission from Mulkey et al., 2017 [73]. (B) EEG epoch from a 6-month-old child with a GoF variant in *KCNQ2* (c.593G>A, p.R198Q), showing modified hypsarrhythmia pattern consisting of generalized background slowing and multifocal epileptiform discharges. With permission from Millichap et al., 2017 [82]. (C) Sleep EEG from a 30-month-old child with a GoF variant in *KCNQ3* (c.689G>A, p.R230H), showing abundant multifocal epileptiform discharges.

vigabatrin in a couple of patients [73]. A similar, if not identical, condition (neonatal encephalopathy, hypotonia, cleft palate, myoclonus, and suppression burst EEG) has been reported with the *KCNQ2*-V175L variant with GoF properties [112].

Infantile Spasms with Hypsarrhythmia

Infantile spasms with hypsarrhythmia, presenting between four and five months of age, without preceding neonatal seizures or encephalopathy is caused by variants that neutralize the first arginine residue in the S4 transmembrane segment of *KCNQ2* (R198Q) [82]. Subsequent neurodevelopmental disability is typically severe (nonverbal and nonambulatory) and MRI shows mild cerebral volume loss. Some may transition to other seizure types. Of note, one patient with epileptic spasms that resolved in response to corticosteroid treatment still had neurodevelopmental delay, but was not as severe as other cases (able to sit and babble at three years), highlighting both the importance and the limitations of rapid successful resolution of infantile spasms in this condition.

In addition, global neurodevelopmental delay and hypotonia without neonatal epilepsy has also been reported for *KCNQ2* substitutions at arginine-144 (R144Q, R144W, R144G) [113–115]. Seizures and/or epileptiform EEG have been reported for some patients, including infantile spasms in a patient with R144Q [113]. MRI shows delayed myelination that resolves or mild ventricular dilatation [115]. Neutralization of this arginine also imparts gain-of-function effects [83].

Intellectual Disability with Sleep-Potentiated Multifocal Spikes

Individuals with *KCNQ3* variants resulting in substitutions at arginine-230 (R230C, R230H, R230S) come to clinical attention as a result of global developmental delay that manifests during the first or second year of life [111]. Most children learn to walk, but language is usually profoundly affected and individuals are nonverbal or limited to a few words. Problematic behaviors and autistic symptoms are common, and many children are diagnosed with autism spectrum disorder. Brain MRIs are usually normal or show mild nonspecific abnormalities.

A minority of patients develop seizures, but many patients get EEGs for staring episodes. Most EEGs recorded between 1 and 10 years of age show spikes with a focal or multifocal distribution, usually potentiated during sleep (**Fig. 15c**). The abundance of spikes in sleep can be near-continuous, raising concerns for epileptic encephalopathy [111]. It is unclear to what extent behavior or cognition might be improved by suppressing abundant spikes in sleep. Response may be seen to high-dose benzodiazepine treatment.

The causative de novo variants in *KCNQ3* neutralize the first two arginine residues in the S4 transmembrane domain and so are paralogues of the *KCNQ2* variants responsible for the neurodevelopmental disability with neonatal myoclonic encephalopathy and/or infantile spasms described above (*KCNQ3*-R230 ~ *KCNQ2*-R201 and *KCNQ3*-R227 ~ *KCNQ2*-R198). *KCNQ3* GoF variants were identified in cohorts sequenced for epilepsy, intellectual disability, autism, and cortical visual impairment, suggesting that these recurrent mutations make an important contribution to the genetic landscape of these conditions. Patients with *KCNQ3*-R227Q appear to have a similar but milder phenotype (e.g., moderate intellectual disability but able to speak in sentences), though relatively fewer patients have been reported [111].

Neurodevelopmental disability resulting from GoF variants in *KCNQ2* and *KCNQ3* spans a spectrum of clinical severity, ranging from profound impairment with even central control of respiration compromised to moderate intellectual disability. The severity of neurodevelopmental disease is generally paralleled by the age at which patients come to clinical attention (**Fig. 16**), ranging from the neonatal period, to infancy, to the second year of life. This in turn is associated with age-related epileptiform EEG abnormalities, ranging from burst-suppression, to hypsarrhythmia, to abundant sleep-potentiated spikes.

Gain-of-function Genotypes and Phenotypes

	KCNQ2 R201C/H KCNQ2 V175L	KCNQ2 R198Q KCNQ2 R144Q	KCNQ3 R230C/H/S KCNQ2 R144G/W	KCNQ3 R227Q
Age of presentation	<1 month	4–6 months	1st or 2nd year of life	2nd year of life
Electroclinical phenotype	neonatal encephalopathy, myoclonus, hypoventilation, suppression-burst EEG	infantile spasms, hypsarrhythmia	intellectual disability, ± autism, ± epilepsy, ± epileptiform EEG	intellectual disability, ± autism, ± epileptiform EEG
Neurodevelopmental impairment	Profound	Severe	Moderate-severe	Moderate

Figure 16 Genotypes and phenotypes of gain-of-function (GoF) variants in *KCNQ2* and *KCNQ3*. Age of presentation is associated with the severity of electroencephalography (EEG) abnormalities and neurodevelopmental outcomes. For GoF variants in the S4 transmembrane domain of the voltage sensor, *KCNQ2* variants impart more severe phenotypes than paralogous *KCNQ3* variants (*KCNQ2* R201 variants are more severe than *KCNQ3* R230 variants, and *KCNQ2* R198 variants are more severe than *KCNQ3* R227 variants). Within each channel, variants affecting the second arginine impart more severe phenotypes than those affecting the first arginine (for *KCNQ2*, R201 variants are more severe than R198 variants; for *KCNQ3*, R230 variants are more severe than R227 variants).

Mosaicism

Special mention should be made of mosaicism, which results from post-zygotic mutation leading to the presence of a pathogenic variant in some proportion but not all of an individual's cells. Mosaic variants are typically associated with less severe disease. The possibility of parental germline mosaicism has critical implications for counseling families on the risk of recurrence of apparently sporadic epilepsy and/or neurodevelopmental disability due to *KCNQ2* or *KCNQ3* pathogenic variants.

Treatment of *KCNQ2*- and *KCNQ3*-Related Epilepsies

The treatment of *KCNQ2*-associated epilepsies has a twofold aim: to achieve seizure freedom, and to normalize, improve, and prevent the severe cognitive and behavioral impairment associated with DEE. Ideally, a treatment should be effective on both seizures and neurodevelopment, and research is moving in this direction. However, for many DEEs, including KCNQ2-DEE, this goal has not yet been realized. In this section, we will address the treatment of seizures in patients with both self-limiting and DEE forms of *KCNQ2*- and *KCNQ3*-associated epilepsy and discuss emerging precision medicine strategies and investigational drugs for the treatment/prevention of the cognitive impairment. The ultimate goal is to provide patients with the best available treatment for seizures, and opportunities for disease-modifying therapies. This perspective holds the promise to intervene with the disease process to prevent or reduce the damaging effects on the developing brain that have taken place.

Treatment of Seizures in *KCNQ2*- and *KCNQ3*-Associated Epilepsies Due to LoF Variants

Historically, in neonates, different types and etiologies of seizures are lumped together and labeled as "neonatal seizures," and treatment relies on a one-size-fits-all approach. This strategy has the unfortunate effect of obscuring seizures as heterogeneous manifestations of specific diseases. Drug trials in neonates have been particularly challenging because treatments have been directed to "neonatal seizures" as a whole, without any distinction between therapies for acute symptomatic seizures and neonatal-onset epilepsies. Lumping all seizure types and etiologies together explains the disappointing situation that the treatment of seizures in neonates has remained substantially unchanged for decades [116–118]. More than 90% of neonates with seizures receive high-dose intravenous phenobarbital. Although phenobarbital has unequivocal efficacy in stopping seizures due to hypoxic-ischemic encephalopathy [119], it is not effective in the majority of neonates with genetic epilepsies, including those associated with *KCNQ2* pathogenic variants [86,87,89,120,121]. In addition, animal studies have shown that even short-term administration of phenobarbital and benzodiazepines increases apoptosis of immature neurons [122–124], impairs cell proliferation, and inhibits neurogenesis in the immature brain [125]. It is essential to dispose of the old monolithic notion of "neonatal seizures," acknowledge that "neonatal seizures" are not a single disease, and recognize that some neonates with acute symptomatic seizures require different treatment approaches [126].

The recognition of the specific seizure phenotype in neonates with *KCNQ2-* associated epilepsies resulted in initial trials of CBZ. For most patients, a dramatic response was observed, with substantial reduction in seizure burden within hours of the first administration of the drug [85,87,89]. Importantly, CBZ is contraindicated in epileptic spasms, the main seizure type of Ohtahara syndrome [127,128]. Subsequently, multicenter retrospective studies confirmed the efficacy of sodium channel blockers on seizures in both SLFNE and DEE associated with KCNQ2 or KCNQ3 variants. Nowadays, sodium channel blockers are considered first-line anti-seizure medications in KCNQ2-related epilepsies associated with LoF variants [85,87,89,129,130]. Although retrospective studies provided support for the use of CBZ in KCNQ2-related epilepsies, there are no prospective randomized controlled studies.

Compared with phenobarbital, CBZ has shown to be well tolerated without the side effects of sedation and hypotension. Thus, it is reasonable to use sodium channel blockers such as CBZ or oxcarbazepine as first-line anti-seizure therapy in patients with *KCNQ2*-associated SLFNE and DEE. Interestingly, some patients with SLFNE may respond to phenobarbital as monotherapy or more often polytherapy [131], but therapy with phenobarbital is mostly ineffective in patients with KCNQ2-DEE and it is not recommended in this setting.

Sodium channel blockers impair the conduction of sodium ions through the channels, suppress repetitive firing, and block the development of seizures [132]. Voltage-gated sodium channels and KCNQ potassium channels co-localize at the neuronal membrane [133]. Therefore, a modulating effect of sodium channel blockers on both sodium and potassium channels has been suggested [89].

As discussed in the Basic Science section, retigabine (ezogabine) is a selective opener of K_V7 potassium channels. Findings from in vitro functional studies raised hope that retigabine could be a targeted treatment for patients with KCNQ2-DEE associated with LoF pathogenic variants. Although, initially, one patient treated with retigabine was reported with a marked reduction in seizure frequency [102], the only retrospective study showed mixed results [80]. Among patients with KCNQ2-DEE associated with LoF variants, five of nine patients treated with retigabine showed some improvement in seizure frequency. Furthermore, parents or treating physicians reported some improvement in development as well, with a better response in those treated before age five months. However, no patient treated with retigabine had complete seizure freedom. This suggests that early initiation of treatment with retigabine may be beneficial, but case numbers are too small to make definite conclusions. The recent analysis by Kuesten and colleagues could not detect a benefit of retigabine compared to other drugs such as sodium channel blockers [131]. However, response to retigabine may vary by *KCNQ2* variant [77].

Targeted therapies for rare diseases need their efficacy and safety evaluated, but due to the small number of potential trial participants, a standard randomized controlled trial is not feasible without large multinational collaboration. In addition, regarding retigabine, before a more standardized trial could be organized, the drug was withdrawn from the market by the manufacturer. Very recently however, the EPIK trial was launched: a double-blind, placebo controlled randomized trial that will investigate the potential anti-seizure effects of adjunctive XEN496, a new pediatric formulation of retigabine.[6] Primary outcome measures will focus on seizure reduction, but during the treatment period and the subsequent open label extension study, information on quality of life and neurodevelopment will also be collected. Next generation Kv7 activators XEN1101[134,135] and BVH-7000 (formally KB-3061 with improved channel subtype selectivity and greater potency are also proceeding toward clinical trials.

Few studies report treatment response in epilepsies due to LoF variants in *KCNQ3*, which are much rarer compared to *KCNQ2*. Case series show a good effect of sodium channel blockers on seizures in the self-limiting form [87]. On the other hand, very few cases of KCNQ3-DEE have been reported [95,109] with different responses to various anti-seizure medications.

Treatment of Neurodevelopmental Comorbidities of *KCNQ2*-DEE Due to LoF Variants

Over the past few years, several descriptive studies and feedback from parents have highlighted the impact of nonseizure-related disabilities (comorbidities or coexpressions as mentioned in an earlier section) on quality of life of children with KCNQ2-DEE, and have clearly defined patient-relevant outcomes [5,6]. So far however, none of the currently available treatments for KCNQ2-DEE have shown a relevant effect on improving neurodevelopment or counteracting other comorbidities.

Given the evidence of the detrimental effect of frequent seizure activity on the developing brain, early seizure control is expected to lead to better neuro-developmental outcomes [136]. In KCNQ2-DEE, early diagnosis of the disorder and early start of a sodium channel blocker to abolish ongoing seizure activity are therefore essential. However, the heterogeneity in cognitive, language, and motor outcomes associated with KCNQ2-DEE makes it difficult to distinguish the effect of early seizure control from the natural variability in neurodevelopmental outcome in small retrospective studies [6]. It is clear that

---

[6] ClinicalTrials.gov Identifier: NCT04639310.   [7] ClinicalTrials.gov Identifier: NCT03796962.

control of clinical seizures alone is essential but not enough to prevent the development of KCNQ2-DEE. Therefore, there is an unmet need for therapies that can intervene on development and modify the long-term outcome of those infants. Potassium channel activators such as retigabine theoretically hold the promise to directly target the underlying disease mechanism and thus also improve KCNQ2-DEE related comorbidities. Gene editing and antisense oligonucleotide approaches are expected to be evaluated as therapeutic options in the next decade [137–139].

In the retrospective study of Millichap et al. (2016), subjective improvement of development was noted for some children treated with retigabine. However, validated nonseizure related outcome measures sufficiently sensitive to capture meaningful change over time will need to be included in future formal clinical trials to prove such an effect. As in most DEEs, studies of therapeutic outcomes for KCNQ2/3-DEE to date have all focused on seizures, including the EPIK trial that is recruiting only children with frequent ongoing seizures. Secondary outcome measures will include developmental, behavioral, quality of life, and sleep quality scales. Results from this study should be an incentive for other trials with nonseizure related outcome measures, including neurodevelopment, as primary endpoints.

Treatment of *KCNQ2* and *KCNQ3* Phenotypes Associated with GoF Variants

Because of their recent recognition, there are currently no established treatment recommendations for patients with *KCNQ2*- and *KCNQ3*-related disorders associated with GoF variants. Case series are small, and in children who do develop seizures, response to anti-seizure medications is heterogenous. In some children with GoF variants *KCNQ2*-R201C or *KCNQ2*-R201H, spasms and non-epileptic myoclonus seemed to respond to vigabatrin, but this was not a consistent finding [73]. Therefore, drug choices should address the seizure type rather than follow gene-specific treatment guidelines. A recent study of individuals with neurodevelopmental disabilities associated with *KCNQ3* GoF variants reported that most patients have an EEG pattern characterized by abundant sleep-activated spikes up to multifocal status epilepticus during sleep that may contribute to the developmental disorder [111]. Future studies should address whether treatment of the near-continuous epileptic activity during sleep seen in some patients with *KCNQ2* and *KCNQ3* GoF variants may prevent or reverse the neurodevelopmental problems seen in these children.

Abbreviations

AIS	axon initial segment
AKAP	A-kinase-anchoring protein
ASD	autism spectrum disorder
BFNE	benign familial neonatal epilepsy
CaM	calmodulin
CBZ	carbamazepine
CRH	corticotrophin-releasing hormone
DAG	diacylglycerol
DEE	developmental and epileptic encephalopathy
EBN1	epilepsy benign neonatal locus 1
EBN2	epilepsy benign neonatal locus 2
EEG	electroencephalography
EME	early myoclonic encephalopathy
fEPSP	fast excitatory post-synaptic potential
GABA	gamma-aminobutyric acid
GoF	gain-of-function
IP3	inositol trisphosphate
iPSC	induced pluripotent stem cells
KCNQ2	gene encoding the $K_V7.2$ (KCNQ2) neuronal voltage-gated potassium channel
KCNQ3	gene encoding the $K_V7.3$ (KCNQ3) neuronal voltage-gated potassium channel
K_V channels	voltage-gated potassium channels
$K_V7.1$	cardiac voltage-gated potassium channel encoded by *KCNQ1*
$K_V7.2$ (or non-italicized KCNQ2)	neuronal voltage-gated K^+ channel encoded by *KCNQ2*
$K_V7.3$ (or non-italicized KCNQ3)	neuronal voltage-gated $K+$ channel encoded by *KCNQ3*
LoF	loss-of-function
mAHP	medium afterhyperpolarization
MRI	magnetic resonance imaging
mRNA	messenger RNA
NPY/AgRP	neuropeptide Y/agouti gene-related protein
PIP_2	phosphatidylinositol 4,5-bisphosphate
PKA	protein kinase A

PKC	protein kinase C
PLC	phospholipase C
POMC	pro-opiomelanocortin
PTX	pentylenetetrazole
RTN	retrotrapezoid nucleus
sEPSP	slow excitatory post-synaptic potential
SLFNE	self-limited familial neonatal epilepsy
SL(F)NE	self-limited familial and nonfamilial neonatal epilepsy
SLFIE	self-limited familial infantile epilepsy
SLFNIE	self-limited familial neonatal-infantile epilepsy

Appendix

Transcript from Video 1: Interview of Anne Berg, Ph.D. by Sara James

Sara James (SJ): We are joined now by Professor Anne Berg. Professor Berg is with the Ann and Robert H. Lurie Children's Hospital of Chicago and the Northwestern Feinberg School of Medicine, Departments of Pediatrics and Neurological Surgery. Professor Berg, thank you so much for joining us to talk about KCNQ2.

Anne Berg (AB): Thank you for having me, it's a pleasure and an honor.

SJ: We're excited to talk in particular about the natural history project on KCNQ2, which you launched, and that research, that data, is really quite hot off the presses. It just came out in February of 2021, so this year, as you and I are speaking. Can you tell me a little bit more about that? How many families participated?

AB: We had 86 families from around the world, mostly US but we had a smattering across the entire globe. It was a nice participation.

SJ: That is; that's terrific. And what were you looking for in this project?

AB: The purpose of the natural history project is really to address a very important goal in clinical trials design, and that is to understand what kinds of outcomes are important to target when developing and testing new therapies. We always think about KCNQ2 in terms of epilepsy, but I think anyone living with a child who has *KCNQ2*-associated disorder knows that this disorder is far more than seizures alone. The purpose of our study is to try to understand what those other components were, how severe they were, how common they were, how they affected the family, and what was most important to parents.

SJ: It's such an important area of research because, you're right, that is exactly what families always say. Seizures are only part of the picture, and sometimes they're not the main part of the picture. In your research, what did you discover to be some of the most significant issues for parents? Can you play out some of that data for us?

AB: Sure. In terms of just basic function, children with *KCNQ2*-associated disorders often cannot walk. They are nonverbal. They may be noncommunicative; we can be communicative without spoken speech, but many of them can't even communicate with sign language or gestures. They have dysfunction in basic autonomic function; they do not sleep well, they have tremendous GI problems, and then other areas regulated by the autonomic nervous system are often impaired: cardiac, respiration, temperature control. Many children have what's called cortical visual impairment. It used to be called cortical blindness; it's not exactly blindness, but it's a failure of the visual cortex and association cortices to process visual information in a way that we can use effectively. So, really, when you think about a child with KCNQ2 encephalopathy, anything that is regulated by the nervous system may be dysregulated in a child with KCNQ2, and most of these children have many areas that are affected.

SJ: One of the aspects about KCNQ2 that really strikes me from a position of being a parent of a KCNQ2 child and seeing so many of these children at family summits and the like, is the different presentation. Did that pop up in your study as well, that KCNQ2 is quite a situation where each child really is unique, that you see a lot of situations where there are common trends, but children can do pretty well and there really is a range. Did that pop up?

AB: There is a huge spectrum of expression in KCNQ2-related disorder and, in fact, KCNQ2 mutations, as you well know, are also associated with what we call benign neonatal familial epilepsy. And that part of the trick is understanding what kinds of mutations cause more benign type of epilepsy or condition, versus the extraordinarily severe one. And that too is part of natural history, although we've not gotten into the actual variants as much as I would like to. That's going to require a much larger study.

SJ: Does that surprise you in terms of – you study more broadly a lot of different kinds of genetic epilepsy – did you find KCNQ2 to be a bit of an outlier, or different, in terms of other genetic epilepsies which you and your team have also studied?

AB: Actually, that's a great question because we are finding that with everything. We see that with SCN2A, we see that – I could give you an alphabet soup full of genes, but we see very broad expression. And part of the question is, how much of it is the actual variant in the gene versus other factors perhaps in the genome that may be modifying the expression? We don't really know. Right now we're very focused on the monogenic aspect of the disease, but clearly there have to be other factors involved that regulate the expression.

SJ: As you did this research and as it started to pour in from the families, what surprised you as a scientist, or what sort of trends did you look at and say, that is interesting?

AB: We now have the term developmental and epileptic encephalopathy, and we talk about epileptic encephalopathies, the idea being that the seizures are at the root of much of the disability associated with these disorders. Children with KCNQ2 developmental epilepsy and encephalopathy, though, not all of them, but many of them have a very mild seizure course. They can call it mild; I know when the parents are going through it, there's nothing mild about it. But some of these children only have one or two seizures in the neonatal period. In our group that we studied, the seizures were resolved within a year in about half of the children. Most of the kids were seizure free for a few years by the time they were in our study. But that didn't really seem to correlate with how severely impaired they were. So there's much more to the impairment than the seizures alone. And this is critical because, again, we were trying to get some idea of how we might help design randomized trials with meaningful outcomes; and if so many children stop having seizures early on, what is the end point going to be? It has to be something else. So it's just fascinating to see so many of these children not having seizures. In some cases, the seizures have fully resolved and they were off medication. In many cases, they were still on medication and might have seizures if the medications were withdrawn. But it didn't really matter; they still had this tremendous disability.

SJ: Professor Berg, you get to the nub of what we hear from parents, which is: we want to see new treatments, ultimately a cure. We want to see new treatments, new medicines, new protocols that we can use for our children. Given your research, if you were in pharma, if you were a drug company, looking at something to consider as an endpoint other than seizures, what markers might you use based on what your early findings are?

AB: There are many, but I think one of the features of the disease that so many parents find distressing – and this is for parents whose children are affected by KCNQ2 variants but really across the board, with all of these developmental encephalopathies – is the inability to communicate with their child. Having a parent almost break down in tears and say, I don't know if she's hurting, I don't know what's wrong, I don't know if he's hungry, I don't know what to do, I wish he could just tell me. I tell you, if we could improve that – it may not be perfect, but if we could somehow improve the child's ability to communicate verbally or otherwise, that would be phenomenal. So I think you actually will see a lot about studies now looking at features like communication. Behavior is another one. Behavior is tied to communication because some of it ends up being frustration. I can't tell you why I'm in pain so instead I'm going to throw a fit and hit my head against the wall or scratch myself. Kids will do that, too, and it's frustration of being in pain and not being able to say anything and get help for it. These things are all interconnected; they're very, very complex. But I think if we could think about communication and behavior – very important to parents, very important to the people who care for these children – that would probably be a direction to go in. There are other factors, too. Sleep is huge. That of course will affect behavior; if you've ever lost a night's sleep, you know what it does to you.

SJ: We lose a few in this house, Anne!

AB: I bet you do!

SJ: Yes, we hear that from parents.

AB: Sleep is a huge one. So therapies that consider whether or not – or trials that looked at whether or not – the therapy actually improved those sorts of factors might really be very interesting. And a therapy that could improve that, whether or not a child has seizures, would be tremendous.

SJ: Let me ask you another question that comes out of our research on this and looking at it from families. They are curious to know what happens as a child gets older. I'm assuming that in your research you had a range of ages of respondents. Can you tell us the range of ages, and if you noticed any distinctions or differences as an individual with KCNQ2 got older?

AB: Most of the children were actually quite young; over half of them were under five. We only had a few going into the teen years. I'm hesitant to draw too many conclusions from what we have. Older children often tend to look worse, but there's a bias there because KCNQ2 as a genetic cause of a severe disorder was only relatively recently identified. So what we see today, the young ones are diagnosed immediately, right in the NICU. In our hospital, epilepsy panels are sent immediately when you see a baby seizing. An older child, though, a 20-year-old, for example, who has KCNQ2 encephalopathy – when that child was born, there was no genetic testing, and that child has gone through this system that preexisted genetic testing. Some very determined parent said, I am going to find out why this is happening. So we find these highly selected individuals who did finally get tested. The child who had a benign couple of seizures in the neonatal period, seizures resolved, and the child was fine – that child is never going to get tested. So we do see them doing somewhat worse, and that's a real caution about drawing any conclusions from cross-sectional data when we're in rapidly changing times with genetic testing coming in like this.

SJ: I appreciate that cautionary note because I think it's important. And it's a small sample, but nevertheless, Professor Berg, it's a really significant sample because it does tease out what are called comorbidities, a term that kind of strikes fear and trembling into a parent, but really just means the other issues that flank out in a disorder that parents see in their day-to-day lives. Just before we let you go, is there anything else that you can tell us, any statistics or numbers that you'd like to share? We'll have those, of course, separately. Or anything else you want to mention that came out in your important research here?

AB: From the natural history project and also some related studies that we've been doing, which the KCNQ2 community did participate in, it's very clear that we're going to have to do some very careful groundwork in order to find out how best to measure these other aspects. You used the term comorbidity. I like to use the term coexpression, because comorbidity almost sounds like, well, and there's something else. But these are expressions of the same disease and they might be treatable. I like to use that to emphasize that these are aspects of a disorder that could be amenable to change with appropriate therapy. But we really are going to have to focus very carefully on how best to measure things. Just to put that in very simple terms, if you were trying to measure how far, say, an Olympic runner could run in 10 minutes, you would use miles, right? Because they probably can go a few miles or kilometers; let's be more Australian, we can use kilometers. But if you're trying to measure how far a snail can crawl in 10 minutes and you use kilometers, you wouldn't get anywhere. We need to go down to millimeters. So we need to learn how to measure these skills on the millimeter level and not the kilometer level.

SJ: Do you also find as you go through this – I love "coexpressions," by the way, I'm going to take that on from this point forward – as you understand, as we better understand through research the coexpressions and the full way, the global way in which KCNQ2 affects an individual, do you think as we better understand that, we will be better able to come up with further treatments and ways to help individuals with KCNQ2?

AB: Yes, and I think the treatments are going to come first from the laboratory – every now and then some serendipitous finding suddenly becomes a treatment – but most of them are being developed very deliberately. But what's really important is that when they go to trial in humans, we have to be prepared with the right measures. And the problem is that, if we have the wrong measures, our regulatory agencies – and I'm going to bet the Australian one is just as strict as the US one – will say, sorry, your treatment didn't work. The parents might say, oh, he's much better; but if you have the wrong measure, you cannot show it to the FDA or whichever regulatory agency is making the decision. You're out.

SJ: That's a really good point.

AB: As carpenters say, measure twice, cut once. And here we want to measure 10 or 20 times before we go. And it's such a rare disease, we don't have a lot of opportunities. There is one aspect, and I just want to mention it because I think it gets overlooked so much, and that is that KCNQ2 – we think of it as affecting the child, a disease that the child has, but the entire family has it. If the child doesn't sleep, the parents don't sleep. If the child is in crisis, the parent is in crisis. The other siblings don't have the parents that they would like to have and should have. So, I do just want to mention the impact of diseases like KCNQ2 that are horrific on the child him or herself, but they go so far beyond that.

SJ: That is something that we hear from parents so frequently, and I think it's an incredibly important point upon which to finish. Professor Berg, thank you so much for joining us from Chicago. We're delighted you could be part of this Cambridge Elements series.

AB: Thank you for having me. It's great.

Transcript from Video 2: Interviews of parents of KCNQ2-DEE children by Sara James

Seizures

Sara James: KCNQ2 is a genetic epilepsy, so seizures are part of the condition. How significant have seizures been in your son's case?

Mark (Ireland, 8-year-old boy): They're a massive part of our life, to be honest. From day one, the fear of knowing whether Eric will come out of the seizures, are we going to the hospital, what to do, to be trained up and held to your medicines. And even today, he's now eight years old and he's having what we call, I suppose, episodes. We're going in for telemetry EEG. Eric sits, stares, he's lost, there's no – you're not able to intervene in between. You try to calm him. He's nonreactive. And after maybe 5, 10, 15 minutes he will come out screaming and crying. Doctors say they've never seen them before, so we're trying to organize telemetry EEG. It's probably – it is definitely the most worrying part of the condition for us parents. The seizures were clonic-tonic, horrendous; he would stop breathing, very frightening to see. Family members don't want to be on their own with Eric, for obvious reasons. As we speak, we have a nurse downstairs; they come in a couple of hours a week just to give a hand, because we can't even just get ordinary carers in to look after him because of the fear of the seizures and having to intervene on seizures. It's a massive part of life, unfortunately.

Jenny (USA, 3-year-old boy): After my son was born, I believe within three days he started showing seizure activities. It took us a couple months to get the diagnosis because people didn't know what it was, and there was a lot of – and he's also my second child so there's a lot of like, well, your first child is fine so I'm sure this is – it's one of those things that will pass, that kind of thing. I would say, yes, every aspect of our lives has been touched and changed for us. I couldn't agree more. It takes a lot of preparations to go anywhere, to do things, so it made definitely life very, very complicated in a way, and similarly affecting our firstborn in a very similar way; we had his birthday parties in NICU and things like that, because we were in the NICU for quite some time.

Sara James: Are there medical complications? People think about this being a genetic epilepsy and the word epilepsy is in the name. So they think about seizures. But that's the tip of the iceberg, isn't it?

Jenny (USA, 3-year-old boy): Yes, with my son's particular case. Because in the beginning they didn't know exactly what it was that was causing the seizures, he was heavily medicated, which caused him to have respiratory failure. Also eating issues because he had tubes coming out of everywhere so obviously he couldn't – we were trying to breastfeed but he couldn't feed, so he had to be g-tube fed. We're still continuing to deal with the repercussions of some of those treatments we had to go through. Currently he has a trach, whether we think he needs it or not, we're still trying to get evaluated; but it was due to the time he had the respiratory failure. Once again there's a lot of debate on what caused it. And because KCNQ2 is – since people don't know so much about it, everybody's super erring on the cautious side, right? So everybody was very cautious to take maybe some risks in terms of, can we try this? No, because we don't know anything about this we can't, and I don't recommend it. So there was a lot of learning we had to do on our part to say, hey, we're in contact with KCNQ2 families and statistically, yes, kids have low muscle tone, etcetera, but we're not seeing too many kids with too much of a breathing issue, etcetera. So it takes a lot of work on our side and research on our side to work with our medical teams sometimes because people just don't know enough.

Variability

Mark (Ireland, 8-year-old boy): It's a strange condition. A child I know in Italy has Eric's variant, the exact same variant, the chances are one in a billion; and this child is walking and can talk. But yet Eric can't do anything at all. It's just – it's a mind-boggling condition, to be honest.

Communication

Karen (USA, 3-year-old boy): He just started this year to smile, so we love when he gives us his little chuckles and his little smile. He's only laughed a couple of times. So communication is something you have to earn with Nolan. It's not something that anyone can walk into a room and he'll be there and you understand what he's saying or what he intends. It's an earned privilege to understand Nolan's intent and communication through love and attention.

Dimitris (Canada, 12-year-old girl): Obviously I don't think she'll ever talk. It's just not something – she doesn't seem to want to. She has different ways of communicating, but she communicates with us every day. Sometimes it's the gentle pull to what she wants, or pointing to what she wants, and other times it's the uncomfortable communication where she throws stuff because she doesn't like what she's doing or she has a tantrum. But it's all communication. She is stuck in this shell and she wants to get out because she wants to be heard and to be understand. For her, it's frustrating because she doesn't communicate in a way we want her to communicate or we expect her to communicate. And then she does it her own way.

Claire (France, 6-year-old boy): Elliott was born in Australia and we only moved last year, so he spent the first five years of his life in Australia in an English-speaking environment, because his nanny was English, he used to go to day care which was in English, and we spoke French at home. What's mind-boggling to me is – he doesn't speak English any more, although when we left he probably had about 100 words; but if you ask him a question, he'll still say "yes" instead of "oui" very often. But he still understands a lot. So we let them watch TV and it's in English; we read a lot of books; but even songs, like he remembered the words to some English songs. So it's kind of like it's some-where in the back of his mind. Very often for Elliott, it feels like – and I don't know, Mark, if it's been the same for you and Eric – but for us it's been – it really has felt like we need to unlock something and then it's better. We're lucky that Elliott can walk, and it was like this: for a very long time he just was not getting it, he just wasn't getting the concept. And then in a couple of days he was up and running from walking. Communication is the same. It's like he was not speaking and then suddenly he had 20 words, and then he kind of built on that. So it feels like there are blockages in his mind almost. You wouldn't know that he speaks English except if you sing a song he'll know the words, but he won't proactively share that with you.

Autism

Dimitris (Canada, 12-year-old girl): She's also been diagnosed with autism; we got that diagnosis about three or four years ago. For us, it's actually opened up some other avenues of some funding within the province we're in, so it's been beneficial. But it didn't – I mean, it's just another label, it didn't change the way she's growing or what she's doing. Really it helped us because it's kind of a known label in the wide world, so it becomes – it's a label that we can apply and that allows us to apply for more stuff. I was going to say, leverage more resources within the province. Because they look for labels to try to create –

not to create, but it's easy to put things into boxes and apply labels to them and then from a funding perspective or from another perspective to – if I've labeled something, I can try to deal with it in that box.

Sleep

Sara James: What does a child who doesn't sleep look like?

Claire (France, 6-year-old boy): I'm almost cautious of sharing what it is like because I definitely do not want to scare parents. But what it looks like is in a sense similar to what any child who doesn't sleep looks like. We've got another son who doesn't have the disease, and when a child doesn't sleep, it's kind of, you get woken up multiple times a night. The difference with Elliott is that it almost feels like it's out of his control. So we have had episodes where a few times, a few nights a week, he would wake up and just literally scream for like two hours, to a point where my husband and I just had to relieve each other because it's impossible to be near a screaming child for two hours. It's not a scream that another, like newborn or toddler would have. He can't even understand what's happening to him so whether it was nightmares or whatever was going on, just scream nonstop for two hours and then just basically fall asleep of exhaustion. We've had that when he was a bit younger; we've had a few episodes that are like phases, the longest one was about six months where it was happening three, four times a week.

Impact on the Family

Dimitris (Canada, 12-year-old girl): So my daughter was born and started having seizures fairly early in life, three days into her birth so in the neonatal period. Overall, it's greatly affected all of our lives. It's changed really how we view the world, how we live, our day-to-day life. It's been a significant change – it's been very significant in terms of how it's changed just – life becomes different. You have to plan, you have to be more organized. You don't have the luxury of picking up and going on a dime to do anything really, go out for dinner, go to the park becomes a planning event. Life is different.

Kara (USA, 3-year-old boy): KCNQ2 impacted each one of my family members in a very specific, different way. It became my life. It's what I live and breathe every day. His brother had to say goodbye to his mom more than he wanted because Nolan was admitted for the first year and a half of his life every single month, so he had to spend a lot of time without his mom. My husband is a very prideful man who doesn't like to share emotions and has gone very quiet; he's not very descriptive, and he deals much different than me where I've gone totally into what is KCNQ2, what does it do, I need to know it in and out. So when you say has it impacted our lives, it changed our lives. It was my life, and it still is, but different. I'm starting to learn balance, but it took me over three years.

Sara James: What I'm hearing is that there's a before and an after diagnosis; that there's one life that exists up until diagnosis, and then life totally changes. Is that what you're saying?

Kara (USA, 3-year-old boy): Absolutely. It's a different world. It's a different universe I didn't even know existed until Nolan was born. I don't think you know about this world [except], unfortunately, if you're forced to live in it.

Claire (France, 6-year-old boy): We have to plan differently. We always have to have medication with us. We can't just leave him even for 15 minutes with someone who wouldn't know how to administer medication because what if something happens at that time? Even though it doesn't happen frequently, what happens if that's the case? It's always on the back of your mind. It's almost like the chemistry in your brain just changes so you have a little checklist that you run through every time you go outside or every time you put him to bed. I still go and check that he's still breathing. It's awful. Lots of parents don't have to think about that, but we do.

Sara James: What does it feel like to be back at work?

Kara (USA, 3-year-old boy): It's actually nice because I really like my job and I really love my colleagues and I enjoy what I do. For the longest time, I felt like I was nothing more than a mother. And that sounds horrible, but it's true. I lost my identity in every other way. Just when he turned three and we started to get some more stability and we've gotten this private school, I went back to work, am I now feeling more of an identity myself again. So I think going back to work and him going to school actually is good for both of us to become individuals.

The Future

Sara James: Is there a stress of long term?

Jenny (USA, 3-year-old boy): That's been one of my number one top-of-mind since this whole thing happened. After kind of getting over the shock it's like – right now he's small, he's cute, and its manageable in a sense because we're bigger and we're younger. But definitely my husband and I have been discussing long-term solution quite a bit. You're trying to find that balance of not being completely debilitated by it, by the thought of what would happen to my child when I, you know – but at the same time trying to live a fulfilling life and not be consumed by the worry. Because I'm a planner, so I try to plan things ahead. But there are certain things – in that aspect, it is similar to a regular child, any child you have that similar thought, but for our second son it's been a big top-of-mind, so we're starting to think about things already. Do we build out a community for KCNQ2 where families can support each other? We've thought of so many different things and talk about a lot of my life goals starting to evolve around achieving that for him to have a stable and safe future.

Sara James: Is there any one thing that you think people really need to know and understand?

Dimitris (Canada, 12-year-old girl): At the end of the day, my daughter's just a little girl. She's 12 going onto 13 and she's just a little girl like any other little girl out there. She's just a little different.

Jenny (USA, 3-year-old boy): Please get to know our kids. Take the time to get to know them. This is a question I always ask when people, especially doctors, give me their advice on what we should do, etcetera: what would you do if it were your kid? So putting yourselves into our – I know it's going to be really hard to imagine but just put yourself in our shoes and imagine what it would be like, and then think about things from that perspective. Obviously, because there is suffering attached, just physical suffering attached to this disorder, please help us find a cure.

Silver Linings

Mark (Ireland, 8-year-old boy): When Eric was born, the bills coming through the door were horrendous. We were obviously out of work in case Eric passed away, we took some time off, Wendy had to give up work then. We applied for this Medical Card because of the bills. We were told we could fill out this 12, double-sided pages of what you had for breakfast, what you earn, what did you do in the shops. We obviously got refused in the end because the threshold is so low. Like the mad Irish man I am, I decided that this wasn't good enough and any parent going through what we were going through should never, ever, ever have to fill out a form while sleeping on a hospital floor. So we decided, you know what? Let's stand outside government buildings. Let's make this known. We got the media involved. We got politicians involved. We spent 1,057 days outside the gates of government buildings. We got invited in, we'd done every single media channel in Ireland. And four years ago in March, we got the 1970 Health Act that mandates that every child with additional needs in Ireland has free healthcare. So it's been a journey. We were told we couldn't do it. The leader of the country told me there's no way it can happen. And 1,057 days later, every disabled child in Ireland has free healthcare. Thanks to the little man downstairs, I suppose, Ireland has really improved, yes.

Transcript from Video 3: Interview of David Brown, Ph.D. by Sara James

Sara James [SJ]: It is my pleasure to introduce David Brown, Professor of Pharmacology at University College London. Thank you so much for joining us, Professor Brown.

David Brown [DB]: Not at all, not at all. It's fine.

SJ: It is indeed a pleasure to talk to you because there is a significant aspect that relates to KCNQ2 that you can help us understand. Simply, what is the M-current?

DB: It's a little current, but it's proportionally quite big. It's a potassium current which is turned on when a cell is depolarized, when a cell is active. When it's turned on, it dampens down the cell's activity and brings it back to where it started. And then when the cell is repolarized and comes back, this current is switched off. So the current is switched on about 5 or 10 percent at rest, and then it's increasingly switched on as the cell is activated, as it fires action potentials, impulses, they switch more on. That turns the cell off and quiets it down again.

SJ: What is the significance of the M-current?

DB: Well, the significance really is that it controls the behavior of the cell. We're looking at it here from the point of view of epilepsy, and when the current is activated, it's dampening down the chances of epilepsy. And if you block the current, or if there's a mutation of the current or of the channel that's carrying the current, then you have an increased chance of epilepsy. So, in that sense, in epilepsy, that's what's happening. But with other cells which don't show any epileptiform behavior, just the normal things that cells do, it still has a dampening-down effect. When it's switched on, it controls the number of impulses the cell fires, and acts as a sort of braking current. Not emergency-braking current, but a graded-braking current. It controls the activity and excitability of the cell.

SJ: How did the discovery of the M-current come about?

DB: It came about originally from some experiments we were doing on neurons in the sympathetic nervous system, in the peripheral nervous system, starting from mammals, rats. We noted that when you stimulate the input to these cells, the afferent input from the spinal cord, the cells – you fire an electrical shock at them and you get an action potential; and that's well known and has been described in 1913, so that was a long way back. Then after this, if you have a long stimulus of one second or so, you begin to get more impulses. And when we noticed this, the extra impulses were due to the effect of the neurotransmitter released onto these neurons, which is acetylcholine, acting firstly on nicotinic type of receptors to give you the single action potential impulse; and then it's acting on muscarinic receptors, giving you this burst of action potentials. And so our question, really, at that point is, why does stimulating these muscarinic receptors give us this repetitive firing? And we saw this originally when we were working in London, Andy Constanti and I, and the key thing we wanted to find out was why the cell – it was known that the cell would depolarize, from previous work – but why was this associated with this excessive firing? It's impressive listening to it. Unfortunately, I've lost an old sound recording, but if you're stimulating the cell with a little electric pulse, as you give it, say, a little one-second electric pulse, normally speaking you get a little BLIP-BLIP-BLIP-BLIP, just one pulse. But if you stimulate the muscarinic receptors with a long pulse, you get BLIP-BLIP-BLIP-BLIP-BLIP-BLIP-BLIP- BLIP-BLIP-BLIP-BLIP-BLIP-BLIP, like that; and then you switch it off again.

SJ: So, when you were with Paul Adams working in the lab, and you had an opportunity to actually hear this distinctive sound, this quite different sound, what was that moment like for you as a scientist in the lab, starting to understand the M-current?

DB: Well, it was always exciting to us because you've only got this in healthy cells which you hadn't damaged by impaling through too crude a microelectrode. You had to use a very fine microelectrode to not damage the cell, not make the cell leak out all its contents. And if you did that, you only got the single pulse. But if you got a good, healthy cell, you'd get these multiple pulses. And so it was always nice to hear the multiple pulses; you'd say, good, healthy cell, now we can work! Now the problem with doing the work originally on the sympathetic neurons in mammals was the cells are very small and you can't work very hard or do many experiments on them. When I teamed up with Paul Adams, we started to use bullfrog sympathetic neurons. The mammalian ones are about 25–30 micrometers in diameter. The bullfrog ones are about 50–60 micrometers in diameter. So you could get two electrodes into the same cell, and then you could do what they call voltage clamp. You could suppress action potentials and just control the membrane voltage, and then measure the currents firing at different membrane voltages. And that's how we discovered the current itself, by voltage clamping in bullfrog neurons.

SJ: And when you discovered the current itself, what did that look like? In other words, when you discovered what you call the M-current, what did that actually look like? How was that reflected?

DB: It's reflected by a slowly increasing outward current as you depolarize the ganglion cell and get a slowly increasing outward flow of current across the cell membrane. It takes about 100 milliseconds or so to completion and then stays constant – given the second voltage that stays constant for the rest of it. The idea of the voltage is that the faster it comes on, the bigger it is, so you get this sequence of increasing currents.

SJ: Could you explain for me in terms of what that means in an animal, be it a bullfrog or a human? What was the significance for a lay person like me, as a parent and a journalist, what was the significance of what you had discovered with the M-current for what would be happening in an animal?

DB: Well, the M-current itself is continually acting as a brake. So the whole point of it is to suppress excitability, suppress hyperexcitability. But what is important from the animal's point of view is, when you release a transmitter like acetylcholine acting on these muscarinic receptors, you suppress the current or reduce it. That means you reduce its feedback, its braking action to reduce the current, and that allows the cell to be much more excitable. So you get multiple firing instead of single firing when it's being activated. And, essentially, we thought of that current – not having anything to do with epilepsy – we thought of it as a current which is there all the time keeping everything under control, and you selectively inhibit it with a chemical release from some other nerve; selectively inhibit it as an attention-seeking device. In other words, now the cell is getting an impulse coming through the pathway which normally we ignore, but now suddenly it has to take notice of this information it's getting, which is firing repetitively. So it's seeking attention. I first tried to explain this to students, I looked at it this way, because it's present in sensory neurons as well: I was standing there and I said, well, it's like this; it's attention seeking. I'm standing here and I suddenly think, did I put my trousers on this morning? And I'll say, yes, I can feel them. So normally you can't feel your trousers, you're used to standing in them all the time. So any information coming through telling you about the touch from your trousers is suppressed by this type of current. You switch this current off selectively when you think about it – you switch it off and, lo and behold, you can feel your trousers again! You don't have to look down to find out if you have them on. To be honest, we thought more in terms of cognition and attention rather than epilepsy. In other words, it's the ability of a cell to draw attention to something, to information it's receiving, which is the key to us in terms of its physiological function, more a question involving cognition. The story of epilepsy came entirely separately afterwards. The epilepsy story didn't really come through until the first drug selectively to block the M-current came through, which was linopirdine; that was about 1996, which was before the KCNQ2 was known. So before the clones, before the gene for the channel subunits, that was introduced as a cognition enhancer. But it was limited by the fact that if you gave too much, we got epileptic attacks, serious epilepsy. And that was, I think, the first indication that the current might control epilepsies. It came through eventually; a few years later, they had another drug which actually enhanced the current, retigabine, acting as an effective anti-epileptic drug.

SJ: What is the specific role of the M-current and the significance of the M-current when it comes to KCNQ2 encephalopathy?

DB: The two subunits were discovered, KCNQ2 and KCNQ3. KCNQ2, if you like, is the working piece of the channel, and KCNQ3 holds it all together. When it mutated, the current wasn't flowing, that's the trouble.

SJ: That's exactly what I want you to explain. So what is it?

DB: In the mutant ones, the channels didn't open and give you a current. That was the trouble. In most cases, there are various things wrong in individual mutations. Sometimes they aren't fast enough, sometimes they don't open at all, sometimes the channels don't even get made. The mutation actually breaks a bit off the gene, the expressed gene components. So several things happen, but basically the channels don't open properly so there's no current or the rate of the current.

SJ: Just as we sum up here, my understanding about your research was that this was sort of, that this began back in the 1970s as basic science, right?

DB: Yes, curiosity.

SJ: This was, you know, a general scientific endeavor. Curiosity. So much of research now is targeted, and specific, and people are going, you know, laser focus on a teeny tiny little question or detail that they want answered. You just had some big general questions. And it turns out that – the area we're in of this big general question turns out to be incredibly significant for a lot of things, especially epilepsy. Was it hard to get this kind of general, I'm-curious-and-just-want-to-look-into-this research funded, Professor Brown?

DB: Oh, yes! Of course, it was, yes. We were doing general nervous system work, and so we had some specific grants from Medical Research Council, and Paul Adams had one from NIH. But to give you an idea, it was difficult to get money, and when we had started the work, we didn't have a computer. And so after the first year, when we'd actually discovered it and we'd brought it to the neuroscience meeting in America in 1979, we applied to the NIH, or Paul did the application, for a computer to do some more work on this, to NIH. And it was turned down, voted nine against and three in favor, saying it was not possible to voltage clamp the bullfrog sympathetic neurons, and they would not give us the money. Eventually, in the second year, he tried again and did get some money.

SJ: Thank you so much, Professor Brown. I really appreciate your time, and congratulations on your discovery with Paul Adams of the M-current. We appreciate your discussing it with us.

DB: Thank you very much. Quite enjoyable.

Transcript from Video 4: Interview of Nanda Singh, Ph.D. by Sara James

Sara James (SJ): It's my pleasure now to be joined by Dr. Nanda Singh, who is the Lab Director at Myriad Genetics in Salt Lake City, Utah. But Dr. Singh, we're going to actually take you on a trip back through time, back to the mid-1990s, when you were a postdoc at the University of Utah in the Department of Human Genetics. Can you just remember for me, as we begin this interview – I'm picturing you as a postdoc – were you young, hungry, thirsty for a really cool discovery?

Nanda Singh (NS): Yeah, I was! I mean, it's a time in your career where you have to make a name for yourself. Mark Leppert was very, very well-known and had these awesome projects in his lab, and he hired me to be a postdoc in his group, and I was so lucky to be hired to be a part of that team.

SJ: When you started there at the University of Utah in the Department of Human Genetics, I want to talk about BFNC. Tell me first of all what that means, and what in particular your task was.

NS: BFNC stands for benign familial neonatal convulsions. What Mark had done, Mark and his group had collected a lot of families and did the groundwork to show that one of the genes that causes BFNC is located on the long arm of chromosome 20. When I joined the group, Mark had narrowed it to a region of about 20 or so genes, and when I joined the group, I needed to figure out which of those 20 genes contained the mutation or mutations that cause BFNC.

SJ: How did you kind of peel away, if you will, the ones that weren't it?

NS: Mark and his team had found an amazing family that had a deletion of part of their genome directly on top of the KCNQ2 gene. That's how Mark was able to narrow it from, really from 20 to a region that – we didn't know how many genes would be in that region, but that really helped to narrow it. And by going after where that deletion was, KCNQ2 is right in the middle of that deletion.

SJ: What was it like to have that discovery? You were the lead investigator on that team. What was it like to narrow it down to that exact gene, to KCNQ2?

NS: Oh, it was really exciting. It was crazy. It was crazy exciting, you know! Yeah, because you're trying to make a name for yourself. You've got all these people competing to find this thing, right? Genetics is a very competitive business, as you can understand. I mean, just – it was crazy, crazy luck, you know!

SJ: What was the thing that finally got you across the line, that finally got you to be able to say, this is it, it's KCNQ2?

NS: What you have to do is – sometimes what you do, when you're working with something called CDNAs, which are codeine sequences, not the patient DNA, is you have a sequence of a small part of the gene. So what you have to do is to get the entire full length of the gene, right? That was the first step. And then the second step is to prove that you can perturb this gene or mutate this gene and see these mutations in these patients. And so we were lucky enough we had about five families, and we started sequencing; after identifying KCNQ2, we needed to show that if these families have BFNC and KCNQ2 is the gene, we need to be finding mutations in all of these families, right? Because sometimes if you find just one mutation, you're not sure is this really the gene, but if you can show it more than once – two, three, four families – that's really good evidence. And so I think we had about five or six families where we found mutations across the gene, in different parts of the gene for KCNQ2, and that's how we knew we had it.

SJ: You're making such an important point because the work on something like this is in the lab, but it's also clinical. It's also with families. Did you ever get a chance to meet any of the families who were directly affected by the research that you'd done in the lab, or was your work purely in that lab environment?

NS: I was lucky enough to be able to go to some patient meeting – the local Epilepsy Foundation of America chapter in Salt Lake City and then the National chapter – I was able to go to those meetings, invited to go give a talk. You would see not necessarily the patients but the moms of the patients, who would ask you questions. It was very, very moving to talk to those parents.

SJ: Do you remember anything in particular that any of the moms said? I'm picturing, as a mom myself, I'm picturing them thanking you for providing an answer, but I don't want to suggest. Is that the kind of stuff they were saying?

NS: Yes. Help me find what's wrong with my daughter, or something like that. It wasn't just with KCNQ2 because we were working on a lot of different epilepsy projects. In a sense, the Q2 project was sort of wrapped up because you knew the gene and you expect drug companies to take it from there to find targets. But we were working on a lot of different epilepsy projects and for some, where parents did not have an answer, they would ask you, can we help you? Do you want blood samples from our family? Can you work on this project? Those are the kind of questions you would get.

SJ: So it could become quite endless because it's as if, there's one answer, now we need to have more. Speaking of finding more answers, that lab was a very busy place in the 1990s and early 2000s. There was another big discovery buried in a similar place. Tell me about what happened there.

NS: Mark and a researcher at San Antonio – I can't think of his name, I'm drawing a blank on it – anyway, he had a BFNC family also, but the family did not map to chromosome 20; it mapped to chromosome 8. And there was only one family that did this. So when we found KCNQ2 we thought, these families look identical, but the gene from one is on chromosome 8, the gene from the other is on chromosome 20. So when we found the chromosome 20 gene, another postdoc in the lab, Carole Charlier, said, you know what? It's going to be a homologue of KCNQ2. We're looking for a homologue of KCNQ2 on chromosome 8. And it turned out to be KCNQ3.

SJ: What was that like?

NS: That was so interesting, to find them both. Of course, Carole found the full length of KCNQ3 and she starting looking for mutations in that gene, and in the family that mapped to chromosome 8, and she did find the mutation there. But really, the next step was trying to figure out: two genes cause the same disorder; are they working together? And it wasn't our group that did that study, there were other groups. In particular I'm thinking of David McKinnon, I think he was at Stony Brook. They are the ones that discovered that the proteins made by these two genes, KCNQ2 and Q3, work together to make a single potassium channel that regulates excitability in the newborn brain.

SJ: What is fascinating about this to me, listening to you talk about this, is, first of all, you have the world of the lab, the Department of Human Genetics at that time at Utah. And I've seen this happen with scientists before when they're side by side. There is, it seems to me, a correlation with proximity and serendipity. Have you found that? Do you think that what was part of what happened with this kind of back-to-back KCNQ2/KCNQ3, with the two of you working there together in the lab?

NS: Absolutely. We were both young postdocs, really excited, looking for cool things. It was Mark that really gave us both these projects and gave us the tools. Carole and I worked well together. We had independent projects and we started working in parallel, and that's really the best scenario. And that department, the Human Genetics Department, had a history of identifying some amazing genes. So we were walking in the footsteps of people who had done amazing work before we got there, for APC and all these other big genes.

SJ: So it's already a place with a lot of energy and a lot of excitement for that kind of thing. You're giving me a sense of it and a feeling of it. When you got that discovery and you looked at the companion there with KCNQ2 and KCNQ3, and you talked about the excitability in the brain, can you now just for me give a little bit of a description of what you think your discovery meant and means going forward? That kind of laid the groundwork, didn't it, for this understanding? Can you explain that?

NS: What I felt was important – what we were trying to do – was finding a target, finding what's wrong. But the end game is to find a treatment, right? And you can't discover treatments unless you have a target. And so I felt like with the discovery of these two genes, we gave primarily pharmaceutical companies a particular target to go after in discovering anti-epilepsy drugs. And so I think there were some that were in the discovery phase that they found were ligands to the KCNQ2-Q3 potassium channel, to block this channel from being overexcited.

SJ: And as you fast-forward to where we are now; we're speaking in the end of June in 2021. As you look the landscape now, and the fact that we now know that KCNQ2 is a mutation that can have global ramifications for an individual: do you think that your research and the coming research can also help us on the path forward to discover better treatments, not just for seizures but for the entire array of challenges that somebody with KCNQ2 or KCNQ3 faces?

NS: I think so. I think when you discover a gene, it's just barely the beginning. You don't know what it's doing in the brain, all the different things it can be doing, all the different places in the brain it's being expressed, at different times of development and during adulthood – childhood and adulthood, where it's being expressed. So much remains to be done and has been done since then to see what this protein is doing. How do we target it? When do we target it? Those kinds of questions other labs – other investigators have really jumped on those ideas and really run with them.

SJ: I have one final question for you. If you were a – you are now the Lab Director of a big lab in Utah and you're doing different work – if you were giving advice to a young postdoc like yourself who's just getting started and really keen to study more about KCNQ2 and that aspect of genetic epilepsy: what interests you going forward? What do you think deserves more study?

NS: With respect to KCNQ2 or just in general?

SJ: You can do – I never limit scientists, go for it!

NS: I think there are so many childhood disorders, things like autism, or even disorders of the elderly that have a genetic component. I actually ended up, after leaving the University of Utah, I did a fellowship in clinical genetics and I'm boarded in genetics now. That's the thing; you can empower patients by getting a genetic understanding of what's causing their disorders. And there are the big ones out there. It's a very fruitful area for any young postdoc looking for something unique and crazy to go after; there's so much out there. I can just see these grad students coming out of these programs and saying, oh my gosh, you have to work on this! Working on the brain, working on genetic disorders of the brain, I think it's an amazing field. It needs sharp researchers and I think there are a lot of them out there.

SJ: It has been such a pleasure to talk to you, Dr. Singh. Thank you so much for joining us to talk about KCNQ2 and BFNC.

NS: You're welcome, thank you so much. It's been a pleasure.

Transcript of Video 5: Panel Discussion of Researchers Who Study KCNQ2 Biology

Panelists

Edward C. Cooper, M.D. Ph.D., Associate Professor of Neurology, Neuroscience, and Molecular & Human Genetics, Baylor College of Medicine, Houston, TX

Maurizio Taglialatela, M.D. Ph.D., Professor of Pharmacology, Division of Pharmacology, Department of Neuroscience, University of Naples Federico II, Italy

Anastasios Tzingounis, Ph.D., Professor of Neurophysiology and Neurobiology, Department of Physiology and Neurobiology, University of Connecticut, Storrs, CT

Moderator

Alfred L. George, Jr., M.D., Professor and Chair, Department of Pharmacology, Northwestern University Feinberg School of Medicine, Chicago, IL

Al George (AG): Hello, I'm Al George, Professor and Chair of the Department of Pharmacology at the Feinberg School of Medicine at Northwestern University in Chicago. I'm also Deputy Editor of the Cambridge Elements series on Genetics in Epilepsy, and it's my pleasure today to moderate a panel discussion on basic science research related to KCNQ2, the theme of this issue. With me are three scientists who have devoted a considerable amount of time and effort over the past several years to investigating fundamental aspects of KCNQ2 biology, physiology, and pharmacology, and to understand their contributions to epilepsy. I will let each of them go ahead and introduce themselves, and then we'll begin our discussions.

Ed Cooper (EC): I'm Ed Cooper. I'm Associate Professor of Neurology, Neuroscience, and Molecular and Human Genetics at Baylor College of Medicine in Houston, Texas.

Anastasios Tzingounis (AT): Hi, I'm Tasso Tzingounis. I'm a Professor of Neurophysiology and Neurobiology at the University of Connecticut at Storrs, Connecticut.

Maurizio Taglialatela (MT): My name is Maurizio Taglialatela, and I'm a Professor of Pharmacology at University of Naples Federico II in Italy.

AG: Wonderful. Thank you for joining me. The first question I would like to ask the three of you is, what got you interested in studying KCNQ2 in the beginning? Maybe I'll let Maurizio lead off with that question.

MT: There is an anecdote which I would like to tell you about to get started, because I had just come back from the United States after five years of postdoc at Baylor College of Medicine. I was establishing my own lab when a colleague called that he was following a family with benign familial neonatal seizures. They just discovered what the genetic causes were in that family, and they Googled in PubMed, at that time, potassium channels and Naples, and my name came out. So he just decided to call me and say, would you like to join in and study these channels? That's what really got me started on KCNQ2 channels after long, many postdoc years working on other potassium channels.

AG: So, to some extent, KCNQ2 found you?

MT: That's correct, they hunted me.

AG: That's great. Ed, how did you get interested in this?

EC: Serendipity was also involved. At the time I was still a postdoc and working in the laboratory of Lily Jan at UCSF, a distinguished neurophysiologist who had cloned the first potassium channels a few years earlier. Lily was asked to write an editorial, a news-and-views, when the Leppert group, led by Nanda Singh, also participating in this Series, had cloned KCNQ2 and KCNQ3 at the two loci for benign familial neonatal convulsions, as it was called then. Lily asked me if I would help her with some of the clinical angles for her editorial, and actually I built a figure that appears in the Journal, accompanying the articles, which was uncredited. But nonetheless, she turned me on to the idea of working on this channel which had a direct role in human disease, and that was a wonderful opportunity I am forever grateful for.

AG: A good example of being in the right place at the right time.

EC: Indeed.

AG: Tasso, how did you get started?

AT: My initiation to the KCNQ2 channel field was coincidental. I was a postdoc at UCSF working with Roger Nicoll, who's also a renowned neurophysiologist. Part of my project was to identify the molecular components of another potassium current, calcium-activated potassium channel. During the course of my studies, it turns out that KCNQ2 channels probably mediate some component of this process, and this is how we all started. Then the more we did the work on it, the more I got interested in KCNQ2 channels, and I continued working on them as a faculty after my postdoc.

AG: Great, thank you. Given that most of you have now worked on KCNQ2 for more or less about two decades, I'm interested in knowing what continually motivates you to keep studying this? Ed, I think you've been probably in this as long as anyone, so what is your continual motivation for working on KCNQ2?

EC: This topic has been a source of ongoing renewal in terms of the source of interest. I would have to say for the last decade or so, the primary motivation has been, came, from the discovery of seriously ill children affected by variants in KCNQ2 and later KCNQ3. There's also really an enormous amount of basic biological interest, which is also mirrored in the deficits that some children have. So these channels are involved in our ability to think, our ability to speak, our ability to control and learn to control our bodies during development. And all of those things are of tremendous interest, of course.

AG: That's great. Let's go to Tasso; what is motivating you to keep studying KCNQ2?

AT: I found the biology very unique and very fascinating. I think we have just started to scratch its biology. What makes this channel so unique? The human body has about 70 potassium channels, depending on how you count, yet only KCNQ2 and KCNQ3 channels lead to very severe disorders. What makes them so special? That's really my interest. And now more recently, the human component of course is very important, trying to understand how the neurons change their properties when KCNQ2 channel is mutated. It's a fascinating question to me.

AG: So a lot of fundamental biology and physiology that ties in with KCNQ2 that we don't completely understand is a great motivator. Maurizio, what is continually motiving you now?

MT: Definitely the pharmacology of this channel is quite fascinating, as both Ed and Tasso introduced. The multiplicity of roles that these channels play give us the opportunity to intervene pharmacologically with drugs. And we have already examples of drugs that have been effective in treating some specific neuropsychiatric disorders. But there is a huge possibility for improvement of these drugs, and that is what I'm trying to contribute to.

AG: That's great. Given that there's still a lot that we don't know, maybe each of you could comment, maybe we could have a little discussion about what are the areas where there is a gap in knowledge related to KCNQ2 that we should be focused on? And what is your opinion about what are those important gaps in our knowledge right now? Let me throw it to Tasso to begin.

AT: I think one of the biggest gaps is, we still don't understand how the loss of function of KCNQ2 as well as the gain of function of KCNQ2 lead to disease, and how do they both change excitability, in some ways similarly but in many ways also differently. We still have no mechanism to understand the gain of function that happens; some ideas out there, but nothing has been yet tested.

MT: I think that the main challenge here for a disease that expresses itself so early in life is that it provides a unique opportunity to disentangle the contribution of epilepsy to neurodevelopment. And that is quite a relevant issue also, if we consider that in order to affect the neurodevelopmental trajectory, we need early intervention. So, how early is this intervention? Do we have a time window opportunity to intervene? Those are the critical questions, at least in my view, that will affect the patient's life in the near future.

AG: I think, Ed, you probably have some ideas about developmental evolution of these conditions and expression of the channel.

EC: Yes. I think that, working with the children and their families, we see that the disease is manifest in different ways at different stages of development. Although we've made great progress in the past decade in understanding some of the molecular changes associated with variants – in effect the molecular pathophysiology at the level of the circuit and how that circuit is linked to behavior during the stages, the miraculous stages of human development – those are areas where we have so much to learn. I think we have some opportunities to make progress moving forward as well.

AG: I think Maurizio said it best; whether we can learn enough to understand the optimal timing of intervening to treat children who have the severe forms of KCNQ2 encephalopathy is a really good point. Do we know enough even now about the disease or the physiology to even address that? I'd say that's a great open question.

MT: We are also developing the right tools to address those questions. I think that's very informative. The KCNQ2 field is providing some valuable information for many other fields. That's what we like about being in this group.

AG: Any other comments, gentlemen? Go ahead, Ed.

EC: I agree. I think that some of the work going on in our laboratories and other laboratories that's relatively new – developing models based on human stem cells or based on animal models – allows us to now begin to dissect these questions in much greater detail and build on the work that we've completed over the last few years.

AT: I agree. I also think one of the challenges is, we don't know if we re-express KCNQ2 channels later in life, will it manage to rescue some of the phenotypes? Is it going to remodel the brain back to a state that is much more feasible for the patient's quality of life? I think one of the challenges is that the KCNQ2 channels have very large proteins; they're very large, so it's difficult to create tools to reintroduce it as well. So I think you need technologies also that will be able to be optimized for KCNQ2 channels specifically. It's not simple to just take technologies from other fields and adapt it immediately. It requires some fine-tuning, and I think we're at the very beginning of that.

AG: I think a lot of things we've discussed today are really emphasizing the important role that basic science and basic research discoveries have had on propelling fields related to human disease. I think KCNQ2 is a great example of that. All of the work the three of you have contributed to, I think, is a testament to that. Also, similarly, the motivating factor of knowing that there's a child out there that has this disease, and the urgency of trying to understand the biology of the gene and the ion channel that it produces is really important. Any last words, gentlemen? Maurizio?

MT: What we can say is that we have the feeling that we are just contributing to a much larger effort, and the great interest that we have in this field is because we see it very translational. Also, in our collaborative efforts, I have to say that these transpire quite clearly, that we go from the basic biology all the way to understanding a little bit better of the clinical, and hopefully also of the treatments of this gene.

EC: I agree.

AT: Fully agree.

AG: I think we'll wrap there. Thank you all for joining me today. I look forward to speaking to all of you in the future.

References

1. A. H. Poduri, A. L. George, Jr., E. L. Heinzen, D. Lowenstein, S. James, *How we got to where we're going*, A. H. Poduri, ed. (Cambridge: Cambridge University Press, 2021).

2. N. A. Singh, C. Charlier, D. Stauffer et al., A novel potassium channel gene, KCNQ2, is mutated in an inherited epilepsy of newborns, *Nat Genet*, 18 (1998), 25–9. DOI: https://doi.org/10.1038/ng0198-25.

3. C. Charlier, N. A. Singh, S. G. Ryan et al., A pore mutation in a novel KQT-like potassium channel gene in an idiopathic epilepsy family, *Nat Genet*, 18 (1998), 53–5. DOI: https://doi.org/10.1038/ng0198-53.

4. A. S. Lindy, M. B. Stosser, E. Butler et al., Diagnostic outcomes for genetic testing of 70 genes in 8565 patients with epilepsy and neurodevelopmental disorders, *Epilepsia*, 59 (2018), 1062–71. DOI: https://doi.org/10.1111/epi.14074.

5. A. T. Berg, D. Gaebler-Spira, G. Wilkening et al., Nonseizure consequences of Dravet syndrome, KCNQ2-DEE, KCNB1-DEE, Lennox-Gastaut syndrome, ESES: a functional framework, *Epilepsy Behav*, 111 (2020), 107287. DOI: https://doi.org/10.1016/j.yebeh.2020.107287.

6. A. T. Berg, S. Mahida, A. Poduri, KCNQ2-DEE: developmental or epileptic encephalopathy? *Ann Clin Transl Neurol*, 8 (2021), 666–76. DOI: https://doi.org/10.1002/acn3.51316.

7. V. C. Beck, L. L. Isom, A. T. Berg, Gastrointestinal symptoms and channelopathy-associated epilepsy, *J Pediatr*, 237 (2021), 41–9.e1. DOI: https://doi.org/10.1016/j.jpeds.2021.06.034.

8. D. A. Brown, Neurons, receptors, and channels, *Annu Rev Pharmacol Toxicol*, 60 (2020), 9–30. DOI: https://doi.org/10.1146/annurev-pharmtox-010919-023755.

9. D. A. Brown, A. Constanti, Intracellular observations on the effects of muscarinic agonists on rat sympathetic neurones, *Br J Pharmacol*, 70 (1980), 593–608. DOI: https://doi.org/10.1111/j.1476-5381.1980.tb09778.x.

10. D. A. Brown, P. R. Adams, Muscarinic suppression of a novel voltage-sensitive K+ current in a vertebrate neurone, *Nature*, 283 (1980), 673–6. DOI: https://doi.org/10.1038/283673a0.

11. J. F. Storm, Potassium currents in hippocampal pyramidal cells, *Prog Brain Res*, 83 (1990), 161–87. DOI: https://doi.org/10.1016/s0079-6123(08)61248-0.

12. V. Barrese, J. B. Stott, I. A. Greenwood, KCNQ-encoded potassium channels as therapeutic targets, *Annu Rev Pharmacol Toxicol*, 58 (2018), 625–48. DOI: https://doi.org/10.1146/annurev-pharmtox-010617-052912.

13. I. E. Scheffer, S. Berkovic, G. Capovilla et al., ILAE classification of the epilepsies: position paper of the ILAE Commission for Classification and Terminology, *Epilepsia*, 58 (2017), 512–21. DOI: https://doi.org/10.1111/epi.13709.

14. R. Teubel, A. Rett, Neugeborenen Krampfe im Rahmen einer epileptisch belasten Familie, *Wien Klin Wochenschr*, 76 (1964), 609–13.

15. M. Leppert, V. E. Anderson, T. Quattlebaum et al., Benign familial neonatal convulsions linked to genetic markers on chromosome 20, *Nature*, 337 (1989), 647–8. DOI: https://doi.org/10.1038/337647a0.

16. T. B. Lewis, R. J. Leach, K. Ward, P. O'Connell, S. G. Ryan, Genetic heterogeneity in benign familial neonatal convulsions: identification of a new locus on chromosome 8q, *Am J Hum Genet*, 53 (1993), 670–5.

17. C. Biervert, B. C. Schroeder, C. Kubisch et al., A potassium channel mutation in neonatal human epilepsy, *Science*, 279 (1998), 403–6. DOI: https://doi.org/10.1126/science.279.5349.403.

18. P. J. Schwartz, L. Crotti, R. Insolia, Long-QT syndrome: from genetics to management, *Circ Arrhythm Electrophysiol*, 5 (2012), 868–77. DOI: https://doi.org/10.1161/circep.111.962019.

19. C. Kubisch, B. C. Schroeder, T. Friedrich et al., KCNQ4, a novel potassium channel expressed in sensory outer hair cells, is mutated in dominant deafness, *Cell*, 96 (1999), 437–46. DOI: https://doi.org/10.1016/s0092-8674(00)80556-5.

20. M. V. Soldovieri, F. Miceli, M. Taglialatela, Driving with no brakes: molecular pathophysiology of Kv7 potassium channels, *Physiology (Bethesda)*, 26 (2011), 365–76. DOI: https://doi.org/10.1152/physiol.00009.2011.

21. A. Lehman, S. Thouta, G. M. S. Mancini et al., Loss-of-function and gain-of-function mutations in KCNQ5 cause intellectual disability or epileptic encephalopathy, *Am J Hum Genet*, 101 (2017), 65–74. DOI: https://doi.org/10.1016/j.ajhg.2017.05.016.

22. H. S. Wang, Z. Pan, W. Shi et al., KCNQ2 and KCNQ3 potassium channel subunits: molecular correlates of the M-channel, *Science*, 282 (1998), 1890–3. DOI: https://doi.org/10.1126/science.282.5395.1890.

23. W. P. Yang, P. C. Levesque, W. A. Little et al., Functional expression of two KvLQT1-related potassium channels responsible for an inherited idiopathic epilepsy, *J Biol Chem*, 273 (1998), 19419–23. DOI: https://doi.org/10.1074/jbc.273.31.19419.

24. K. Springer, N. Varghese, A. V. Tzingounis, Flexible Stoichiometry: implications for KCNQ2- and KCNQ3-associated neurodevelopmental disorders, *Dev Neurosci*, 43 (2021), 191–200. DOI: https://doi.org/10.1159/000515495.

25. N. Dirkx, F. Miceli, M. Taglialatela, S. Weckhuysen, The role of Kv7.2 in neurodevelopment: insights and gaps in our understanding, *Front Physiol*, 11 (2020), 570588. DOI: https://doi.org/10.3389/fphys.2020.570588.

26. M. Martire, P. Castaldo, M. D'Amico, P. Preziosi, L. Annunziato, M. Taglialatela, M channels containing KCNQ2 subunits modulate norepinephrine, aspartate, and GABA release from hippocampal nerve terminals, *J Neurosci*, 24 (2004), 592–7. DOI: https://doi.org/10.1523/JNEUROSCI.3143-03.2004.

27. M. Martire, M. D'Amico, E. Panza et al., Involvement of KCNQ2 subunits in [3H]dopamine release triggered by depolarization and pre-synaptic muscarinic receptor activation from rat striatal synaptosomes, *J Neurochem*, 102 (2007), 179–93. DOI: https://doi.org/10.1111/j.1471-4159.2007.04562.x.

28. A. K. Friedman, B. Juarez, S. M. Ku et al., KCNQ channel openers reverse depressive symptoms via an active resilience mechanism, *Nat Commun*, 7 (2016), 11671. DOI: https://doi.org/10.1038/ncomms11671.

29. S. P. Aiken, B. J. Lampe, P. A. Murphy, B. S. Brown, Reduction of spike frequency adaptation and blockade of M-current in rat CA1 pyramidal neurones by linopirdine (DuP 996), a neurotransmitter release enhancer, *Br J Pharmacol*, 115 (1995), 1163–8. DOI: https://doi.org/10.1111/j.1476-5381.1995.tb15019.x.

30. K. Rockwood, B. L. Beattie, M. R. Eastwood et al., A randomized, controlled trial of linopirdine in the treatment of Alzheimer's disease, *Can J Neurol Sci*, 24 (1997), 140–5. DOI: https://doi.org/10.1017/s0317167 10002148x.

31. F. Miceli, M. V. Soldovieri, P. Ambrosino, L. Manocchio, I. Mosca, M. Taglialatela, Pharmacological targeting of neuronal Kv7.2/3 channels: a focus on chemotypes and receptor sites, *Curr Med Chem*, 25 (2018), 2637–60. DOI: https://doi.org/10.2174/0929867324666171012122852.

32. I. Szelenyi, Flupirtine, a re-discovered drug, revisited, *Inflamm Res*, 62 (2013), 251–8. DOI: https://doi.org/10.1007/s00011-013-0592-5.

33. V. Jakovlev, U. Achterrath-Tuckermann, A. von Schlichtegroll, F. Stroman, K. Thiemer, [General pharmacologic studies on the analgesic flupirtine], *Arzneimittelforschung*, 35 (1985), 44–55.

34. A. Rostock, C. Tober, C. Rundfeldt et al., D-23129: a new anticonvulsant with a broad spectrum activity in animal models of epileptic seizures, *Epilepsy Res*, 23 (1996), 211–23. DOI: https://doi.org/10.1016/0920-1211 (95)00101-8.

35. C. Rundfeldt, The new anticonvulsant retigabine (D-23129) acts as an opener of K+ channels in neuronal cells, *Eur J Pharmacol*, 336 (1997), 243–9. DOI: https://doi.org/10.1016/s0014-2999(97)01249-1.

36. T. Garin Shkolnik, H. Feuerman, E. Didkovsky et al., Blue-gray mucocu-taneous discoloration: a new adverse effect of ezogabine, *JAMA Dermatol*, 150 (2014), 984–9. DOI: https://doi.org/10.1001/jamadermatol.2013.8895.

37. S. Clark, A. Antell, K. Kaufman, New antiepileptic medication linked to blue discoloration of the skin and eyes, *Ther Adv Drug Saf*, 6 (2015), 15–9. DOI: https://doi.org/10.1177/2042098614560736.

38. C. Ostacolo, F. Miceli, V. Di Sarno et al., Synthesis and pharmacological characterization of conformationally restricted retigabine analogues as novel neuronal kv7 channel activators, *J Med Chem*, 63 (2020), 163–85. DOI: https://doi.org/10.1021/acs.jmedchem.9b00796.

39. C. Bock, A. Link, How to replace the lost keys? Strategies toward safer KV7 channel openers, *Future Med Chem*, 11.4 (2019). DOI: https://doi.org/10.4155/fmc-2018-0350.

40. P. Delmas, D. A. Brown, Pathways modulating neural KCNQ/M (Kv7) potassium channels, *Nat Rev Neurosci*, 6 (2005), 850–62. DOI: https://doi.org/10.1038/nrn1785.

41. J. Zhang, E. C. Kim, C. Chen et al., Identifying mutation hotspots reveals pathogenetic mechanisms of KCNQ2 epileptic encephalopathy, *Sci Rep*, 10 (2020), 4756. DOI: https://doi.org/10.1038/s41598-020-61697-6.

42. J. Sun, R. MacKinnon, Structural basis of human KCNQ1 modulation and gating, *Cell*, 180 (2020), 340–7 e9. DOI: https://doi.org/10.1016/j.cell.2019.12.003.

43. D. L. Greene, N. Hoshi, Modulation of Kv7 channels and excitability in the brain, *Cell Mol Life Sci*, 74 (2017), 495–508. DOI: https://doi.org/10.1007/s00018-016-2359-y.

44. N. Hoshi, M-current suppression, seizures and lipid metabolism: a potential link between neuronal kv7 channel regulation and dietary therapies for epilepsy, *Front Physiol*, 11 (2020), 513. DOI: https://doi.org/10.3389/fphys.2020.00513.

45. B. C. Schroeder, C. Kubisch, V. Stein, T. J. Jentsch, Moderate loss of function of cyclic-AMP-modulated KCNQ2/KCNQ3 K+ channels causes epilepsy, *Nature*, 396 (1998), 687–90. DOI: https://doi.org/10.1038/25367.

46. H. J. Kim, M. H. Jeong, K. R. Kim et al., Protein arginine methylation facilitates KCNQ channel-PIP2 interaction leading to seizure suppression, *Elife*, 5 (2016). DOI: https://doi.org/10.7554/eLife.17159.

47. N. Gamper, O. Zaika, Y. Li et al., Oxidative modification of M-type K(+) channels as a mechanism of cytoprotective neuronal silencing, *EMBO J*, 25 (2006), 4996–5004. DOI: https://doi.org/10.1038/sj.emboj.7601374.

48. M. J. Saganich, E. Machado, B. Rudy, Differential expression of genes encoding subthreshold-operating voltage-gated K+ channels in brain,

J Neurosci, 21 (2001), 4609–24. DOI: https://doi.org/10.1523/JNEUROSCI .21-13-04609.2001.

49. E. C. Cooper, E. Harrington, Y. N. Jan, L. Y. Jan, M channel KCNQ2 subunits are localized to key sites for control of neuronal network oscillations and synchronization in mouse brain, *J Neurosci*, 21 (2001), 9529–40. DOI: https://doi.org/10.1523/JNEUROSCI.21-24-09529.2001.

50. V. C. Galvin, S. T. Yang, C. D. Paspalas et al., Muscarinic M1 receptors modulate working memory performance and activity via KCNQ potassium channels in the primate prefrontal cortex, *Neuron*, 106 (2020), 649–61. DOI: https://doi.org/10.1016/j.neuron.2020.02.030.

51. A. Battefeld, B. T. Tran, J. Gavrilis, E. C. Cooper, M. H. Kole, Heteromeric Kv7.2/7.3 channels differentially regulate action potential initiation and conduction in neocortical myelinated axons, *J Neurosci*, 34 (2014), 3719–32. DOI: https://doi.org/10.1523/JNEUROSCI.4206-13.2014.

52. C. Yue, Y. Yaari, KCNQ/M channels control spike afterdepolarization and burst generation in hippocampal neurons, *J Neurosci*, 24 (2004), 4614–24. DOI: https://doi.org/10.1523/JNEUROSCI.0765-04.2004.

53. N. Gu, K. Vervaeke, H. Hu, J. F. Storm, Kv7/KCNQ/M and HCN/h, but not KCa2/SK channels, contribute to the somatic medium after-hyperpolarization and excitability control in CA1 hippocampal pyramidal cells, *J Physiol*, 566 (2005), 689–715. DOI: https://doi.org/10.1113/jphysiol.2005.086835.

54. H. C. Peters, H. Hu, O. Pongs, J. F. Storm, D. Isbrandt, Conditional transgenic suppression of M channels in mouse brain reveals functions in neuronal excitability, resonance and behavior, *Nat Neurosci*, 8 (2005), 51–60. DOI: https://doi.org/10.1038/nn1375.

55. H. Soh, R. Pant, J. J. LoTurco, A. V. Tzingounis, Conditional deletions of epilepsy-associated KCNQ2 and KCNQ3 channels from cerebral cortex cause differential effects on neuronal excitability, *J Neurosci*, 34 (2014), 5311–21. DOI: https://doi.org/10.1523/JNEUROSCI.3919-13.2014.

56. W. Hu, B. P. Bean, Differential control of axonal and somatic resting potential by voltage-dependent conductances in cortical layer 5 pyramidal neurons, *Neuron*, 99 (2018), 1315–26. DOI: https://doi.org/10.1016/j .neuron.2018.08.042.

57. J. Verneuil, C. Brocard, V. Trouplin, L. Villard, J. Peyronnet-Roux, F. Brocard, The M-current works in tandem with the persistent sodium current to set the speed of locomotion, *PLoS Biol*, 18 (2020), e3000738. DOI: https://doi.org/10.1371/journal.pbio.3000738.

58. Z. Niday, V. E. Hawkins, H. Soh, D. K. Mulkey, A. V. Tzingounis, Epilepsy-associated KCNQ2 channels regulate multiple intrinsic properties

of layer 2/3 pyramidal neurons, *J Neurosci*, 37 (2017), 576–86. DOI: https://doi.org/10.1523/JNEUROSCI.1425-16.2016.

59. J. J. Lawrence, F. Saraga, J. F. Churchill et al., Somatodendritic Kv7/KCNQ/M channels control interspike interval in hippocampal interneurons, *J Neurosci*, 26 (2006), 12325–38. DOI: https://doi.org/10.1523/JNEUROSCI.3521-06 .2006.

60. K. M. Goff, E. M. Goldberg, Vasoactive intestinal peptide-expressing interneurons are impaired in a mouse model of Dravet syndrome, *Elife*, 8 (2019). DOI: https://doi.org/10.7554/eLife.46846.

61. H. Soh, S. Park, K. Ryan, K. Springer, A. Maheshwari, A. V. Tzingounis, Deletion of KCNQ2/3 potassium channels from PV+ interneurons leads to homeostatic potentiation of excitatory transmission, *Elife*, 7 (2018). DOI: https://doi.org/10.7554/eLife.38617.

62. M. Milh, P. Roubertoux, N. Biba et al., A knock-in mouse model for KCNQ2-related epileptic encephalopathy displays spontaneous general-ized seizures and cognitive impairment, *Epilepsia*, 61 (2020), 868–78. DOI: https://doi.org/10.1111/epi.16494.

63. J. F. Otto, Y. Yang, W. N. Frankel, H. S. White, K. S. Wilcox, A spontaneous mutation involving Kcnq2 (Kv7.2) reduces M-current density and spike frequency adaptation in mouse CA1 neurons, *J Neurosci*, 26 (2006), 2053–9. DOI: https://doi.org/10.1523/JNEUROSCI.1575-05.2006.

64. N. A. Singh, J. F. Otto, E. J. Dahle et al., Mouse models of human KCNQ2 and KCNQ3 mutations for benign familial neonatal convulsions show seiz-ures and neuronal plasticity without synaptic reorganization, *J Physiol*, 586 (2008), 3405–23. DOI: https://doi.org/10.1113/jphysiol.2008.154971.

65. Y. Bi, H. Chen, J. Su, X. Cao, X. Bian, K. Wang, Visceral hyperalgesia induced by forebrain-specific suppression of native Kv7/KCNQ/M-current in mice, *Mol Pain*, 7 (2011), 84. DOI: https://doi.org/10.1186/1744-8069-7-84.

66. D. Simkin, K. A. Marshall, C. G. Vanoye et al., Dyshomeostatic modulation of Ca(2+)-activated K(+) channels in a human neuronal model of KCNQ2 encephalopathy, *Elife*, 10 (2021). DOI: https://doi.org/10.7554/eLife.64434.

67. L. Gautron, J. K. Elmquist, K. W. Williams, Neural control of energy balance: translating circuits to therapies, *Cell*, 161 (2015), 133–45. DOI: https://doi.org/10.1016/j.cell.2015.02.023.

68. M. O. Dietrich, M. R. Zimmer, J. Bober, T. L. Horvath, Hypothalamic AgRP neurons drive stereotypic behaviors beyond feeding, *Cell*, 160 (2015), 1222–32. DOI: https://doi.org/10.1016/j.cell.2015.02.024.

69. T. A. Roepke, J. Qiu, A. W. Smith, O. K. Ronnekleiv, M. J. Kelly, Fasting and 17beta-estradiol differentially modulate the M-current in neuropeptide

Y neurons, *J Neurosci*, 31 (2011), 11825–35. DOI: https://doi.org/10.1523/JNEUROSCI.1395-11.2011.

70. T. L. Stincic, M. A. Bosch, A. C. Hunker et al., CRISPR knockdown of Kcnq3 attenuates the M-current and increases excitability of NPY/AgRP neurons to alter energy balance, *Mol Metab*, 49 (2021), 101218. DOI: https://doi.org/10.1016/j.molmet.2021.101218.

71. J. J. Zhou, Y. Gao, T. A. Kosten, Z. Zhao, D. P. Li, Acute stress diminishes M-current contributing to elevated activity of hypothalamic-pituitary-adrenal axis, *Neuropharmacology*, 114 (2017), 67–76. DOI: https://doi.org/10.1016/j.neuropharm.2016.11.024.

72. P. Nappi, F. Miceli, M. V. Soldovieri, P. Ambrosino, V. Barrese, M. Taglialatela, Epileptic channelopathies caused by neuronal Kv7 (KCNQ) channel dysfunction, *Pflugers Arch*, 472 (2020), 881–98. DOI: https://doi.org/10.1007/s00424-020-02404-2.

73. S. B. Mulkey, B. Ben-Zeev, J. Nicolai et al., Neonatal nonepileptic myoclonus is a prominent clinical feature of KCNQ2 gain-of-function variants R201C and R201H, *Epilepsia*, 58 (2017), 436–45. DOI: https://doi.org/10.1111/epi.13676.

74. P. G. Guyenet, D. A. Bayliss, Neural Control of Breathing and CO_2 Homeostasis, *Neuron*, 87 (2015), 946–61. DOI: https://doi.org/10.1016/j.neuron.2015.08.001.

75. K. Li, S. B. G. Abbott, Y. Shi, P. Eggan, E. C. Gonye, D. A. Bayliss, TRPM4 mediates a subthreshold membrane potential oscillation in respiratory chemoreceptor neurons that drives pacemaker firing and breathing, *Cell Rep*, 34 (2021), 108714. DOI: https://doi.org/10.1016/j.celrep.2021.108714.

76. J. D. Symonds, S. M. Zuberi, K. Stewart et al., Incidence and phenotypes of childhood-onset genetic epilepsies: a prospective population-based national cohort, *Brain*, 142 (2019), 2303–18. DOI: https://doi.org/10.1093/brain/awz195.

77. C. G. Vanoye, R. R. Desai, Z. Ji et al., High-throughput evaluation of epilepsy-associated *KCNQ2* variants reveals functional and pharmacological heterogeneity, *JCI Insight*, in press (2022). DOI: https://doi.org/10.1172/jci.insight.156314

78. F. Miceli, M. V. Soldovieri, P. Ambrosino et al., Genotype-phenotype correlations in neonatal epilepsies caused by mutations in the voltage sensor of K(v)7.2 potassium channel subunits, *Proc Natl Acad Sci U S A*, 110 (2013), 4386–91. DOI: https://doi.org/10.1073/pnas.1216867110.

79. G. Orhan, M. Bock, D. Schepers et al., Dominant-negative effects of KCNQ2 mutations are associated with epileptic encephalopathy, *Ann Neurol*, 75 (2014), 382–94. DOI: https://doi.org/10.1002/ana.24080.

80. J. J. Millichap, K. L. Park, T. Tsuchida et al., KCNQ2 encephalopathy: features, mutational hot spots, and ezogabine treatment of 11 patients, *Neurol Genet*, 2 (2016), e96. DOI: https://doi.org/10.1212/NXG.000000 0000000096.

81. A. Goto, A. Ishii, M. Shibata, Y. Ihara, E. C. Cooper, S. Hirose, Characteristics of KCNQ2 variants causing either benign neonatal epilepsy or developmental and epileptic encephalopathy, *Epilepsia*, 60 (2019), 1870–80. DOI: https://doi.org/10.1111/epi.16314.

82. J. J. Millichap, F. Miceli, M. De Maria et al., Infantile spasms and encephalopathy without preceding neonatal seizures caused by KCNQ2 R198Q, a gain-of-function variant, *Epilepsia*, 58 (2017), e10–e5. DOI: https://doi.org/ 10.1111/epi.13601.

83. F. Miceli, M. V. Soldovieri, P. Ambrosino et al., Early-onset epileptic encephalopathy caused by gain-of-function mutations in the voltage sensor of Kv7.2 and Kv7.3 potassium channel subunits, *J Neurosci*, 35 (2015), 3782–93. DOI: https://doi.org/10.1523/JNEUROSCI.4423-14.2015.

84. Z. Niday, A. V. Tzingounis, Potassium Channel Gain of Function in Epilepsy: An Unresolved Paradox, *Neuroscientist*, 24 (2018), 368–80. DOI: https://doi.org/10.1177/1073858418763752.

85. A. L. Numis, M. Angriman, J. E. Sullivan et al., KCNQ2 encephalopathy: delineation of the electroclinical phenotype and treatment response, *Neurology*, 82 (2014), 368–70. DOI: https://doi.org/10.1212/WNL.0000000 000000060.

86. M. C. Cornet, V. Morabito, D. Lederer et al., Neonatal presentation of genetic epilepsies: early differentiation from acute provoked seizures, *Epilepsia*, (2021). DOI: https://doi.org/10.1111/epi.16957.

87. T. T. Sands, M. Balestri, G. Bellini et al., Rapid and safe response to low-dose carbamazepine in neonatal epilepsy, *Epilepsia*, 57 (2016), 2019–30. DOI: https://doi.org/10.1111/epi.13596.

88. A. Vilan, J. Mendes Ribeiro, P. Striano et al., A distinctive ictal amplitude-integrated electroencephalography pattern in newborns with neonatal epilepsy associated with KCNQ2 mutations, *Neonatology*, 112 (2017), 387–93. DOI: https://doi.org/10.1159/000478651.

89. T. Pisano, A. L. Numis, S. B. Heavin et al., Early and effective treatment of KCNQ2 encephalopathy, *Epilepsia*, 56 (2015), 685–91. DOI: https://doi .org/10.1111/epi.12984.

90. F. Miceli, L. Carotenuto, V. Barrese et al., A Novel Kv7.3 Variant in the voltage-sensing S4 segment in a family with benign neonatal epilepsy: functional characterization and in vitro rescue by β-Hydroxybutyrate, *Front Physiol*, 11 (2020). DOI: https://doi.org/10.3389/fphys.2020.01040.

91. B. E. Grinton, S. E. Heron, J. T. Pelekanos et al., Familial neonatal seizures in 36 families: clinical and genetic features correlate with outcome, *Epilepsia*, 56 (2015), 1071–80. DOI: https://doi.org/10.1111/epi.13020.

92. G. M. Ronen, T. O. Rosales, M. Connolly, V. E. Anderson, M. Leppert, Seizure characteristics in chromosome 20 benign familial neonatal convulsions, *Neurology*, 43 (1993), 1355–60. DOI: https://doi.org/10.1212/wnl.43.7.1355.

93. R. A. Shellhaas, C. J. Wusthoff, T. N. Tsuchida et al., Profile of neonatal epilepsies: characteristics of a prospective US cohort, *Neurology*, 89 (2017), 893–9. DOI: https://doi.org/10.1212/WNL.0000000000004284.

94. F. Zara, N. Specchio, P. Striano et al., Genetic testing in benign familial epilepsies of the first year of life: clinical and diagnostic significance, *Epilepsia*, 54 (2013), 425–36. DOI: https://doi.org/10.1111/epi.12089.

95. F. Miceli, P. Striano, M. V. Soldovieri et al., A novel KCNQ3 mutation in familial epilepsy with focal seizures and intellectual disability, *Epilepsia*, 56 (2015), e15–e20. DOI: https://doi.org/10.1111/epi.12887.

96. K. Dedek, B. Kunath, C. Kananura, U. Reuner, T. J. Jentsch, O. K. Steinlein, Myokymia and neonatal epilepsy caused by a mutation in the voltage sensor of the KCNQ2 K+ channel, *Proc Natl Acad Sci U S A*, 98 (2001), 12272–7. DOI: https://doi.org/10.1073/pnas.211431298.

97. L. Blumkin, A. Suls, T. Deconinck et al., Neonatal seizures associated with a severe neonatal myoclonus like dyskinesia due to a familial KCNQ2 gene mutation, *Eur J Paediatr Neurol*, 16 (2012), 356–60. DOI: https://doi.org/10.1016/j.ejpn.2011.11.004.

98. M. V. Soldovieri, N. Boutry-Kryza, M. Milh et al., Novel KCNQ2 and KCNQ3 mutations in a large cohort of families with benign neonatal epilepsy: first evidence for an altered channel regulation by syntaxin-1A, *Hum Mutat*, 35 (2014), 356–67. DOI: https://doi.org/10.1002/humu.22500.

99. M. Milh, C. Lacoste, P. Cacciagli et al., Variable clinical expression in patients with mosaicism for KCNQ2 mutations, *Am J Med Genet A*, 167A (2015), 2314–8. DOI: https://doi.org/10.1002/ajmg.a.37152.

100. A. H. Sadewa, T. H. Sasongko, M.J. Lee et al., Germ-line mutation of KCNQ2, p.R213W, in a Japanese family with benign familial neonatal convulsion, *Pediatr Int*, 50 (2008), 167–71. DOI: https://doi.org/10.1111/j.1442-200X.2008.02539.x.

101. S. Weckhuysen, S. Mandelstam, A. Suls et al., KCNQ2 encephalopathy: emerging phenotype of a neonatal epileptic encephalopathy, *Ann Neurol*, 71 (2012), 15–25. DOI: https://doi.org/10.1002/ana.22644.

102. S. Weckhuysen, V. Ivanovic, R. Hendrickx et al., Extending the KCNQ2 encephalopathy spectrum: clinical and neuroimaging findings in 17 patients, *Neurology*, 81 (2013), 1697–703. DOI: https://doi.org/10.1212/01.wnl.0000435296.72400.a1.

103. H. E. Olson, M. Kelly, C. M. LaCoursiere et al., Genetics and genotype-phenotype correlations in early onset epileptic encephalopathy with burst suppression, *Ann Neurol*, 81 (2017), 419–29. DOI: https://doi.org/10.1002/ana.24883.

104. H. Saitsu, M. Kato, A. Koide et al., Whole exome sequencing identifies KCNQ2 mutations in Ohtahara syndrome, *Ann Neurol*, 72 (2012), 298–300. DOI: https://doi.org/10.1002/ana.23620.

105. M. Kato, T. Yamagata, M. Kubota et al., Clinical spectrum of early onset epileptic encephalopathies caused by KCNQ2 mutation, *Epilepsia*, 54 (2013), 1282–7. DOI: https://doi.org/10.1111/epi.12200.

106. F. Malerba, G. Alberini, G. Balagura et al., Genotype-phenotype correlations in patients with de novo KCNQ2 pathogenic variants, *Neurol Genet*, 6 (2020), e528. DOI: https://doi.org/10.1212/NXG.0000000000000528.

107. S. Boets, K. M. Johannesen, A. Destree et al., Adult phenotype of KCNQ2 encephalopathy, *J Med Genet*, (2021). DOI: https://doi.org/10.1136/jmedgenet-2020-107449.

108. A. Lauritano, S. Moutton, E. Longobardi et al., A novel homozygous KCNQ3 loss-of-function variant causes non-syndromic intellectual disability and neonatal-onset pharmacodependent epilepsy, *Epilepsia Open*, 4 (2019), 464–75. DOI: https://doi.org/10.1002/epi4.12353.

109. K. Kothur, K. Holman, E. Farnsworth et al., Diagnostic yield of targeted massively parallel sequencing in children with epileptic encephalopathy, *Seizure*, 59 (2018), 132–40. DOI: https://doi.org/10.1016/j.seizure.2018.05.005.

110. P. Ambrosino, E. Freri, B. Castellotti et al., Kv7.3 compound heterozygous variants in early onset encephalopathy reveal additive contribution of c-terminal residues to PIP2-dependent K(+) channel gating, *Mol Neurobiol*, 55 (2018), 7009–24. DOI: https://doi.org/10.1007/s12035-018-0883-5.

111. T. T. Sands, F. Miceli, G. Lesca et al., Autism and developmental disability caused by KCNQ3 gain-of-function variants, *Ann Neurol*, 86 (2019), 181–92. DOI: https://doi.org/10.1002/ana.25522.

112. J. Devaux, A. Abidi, A. Roubertie et al., A Kv7.2 mutation associated with early onset epileptic encephalopathy with suppression-burst enhances Kv7/M channel activity, *Epilepsia*, 57 (2016), e87–e93. DOI: https://doi.org/10.1111/epi.13366.

113. Epi4K Consortium, E. P. G. Project, A. S. Allen et al., De novo mutations in epileptic encephalopathies, *Nature*, 501 (2013), 217–21. DOI: https://doi.org/10.1038/nature12439.

114. Deciphering Developmental Disorders Study, Prevalence and architecture of de novo mutations in developmental disorders, *Nature*, 542 (2017), 433–8. DOI: https://doi.org/10.1038/nature21062.

115. L. Mary, E. Nourisson, C. Feger et al., Pathogenic variants in KCNQ2 cause intellectual deficiency without epilepsy: broadening the phenotypic spectrum of a potassium channelopathy, *Am J Med Genet A*, 185 (2021), 1803–15. DOI: https://doi.org/10.1002/ajmg.a.62181.

116. A. I. Bartha, J. Shen, K. H. Katz et al., Neonatal seizures: multicenter variability in current treatment practices, *Pediatr Neurol*, 37 (2007), 85–90. DOI: https://doi.org/10.1016/j.pediatrneurol.2007.04.003.

117. H. C. Glass, R. A. Shellhaas, C. J. Wusthoff et al., Contemporary profile of seizures in neonates: a prospective cohort study, *J Pediatr*, 174 (2016), 98–103.e1. DOI: https://doi.org/10.1016/j.jpeds.2016.03.035.

118. M. Vento, L. S. de Vries, A. Alberola et al., Approach to seizures in the neonatal period: a European perspective, *Acta Paediatr*, 99 (2010), 497–501. DOI: https://doi.org/10.1111/j.1651-2227.2009.01659.x.

119. C. Sharpe, G. E. Reiner, S. L. Davis et al., Levetiracetam versus phenobarbital for neonatal seizures: a randomized controlled trial, *Pediatrics*, 145 (2020). DOI: https://doi.org/10.1542/peds.2019-3182.

120. T. Maeda, M. Shimizu, K. Sekiguchi et al., Exacerbation of benign familial neonatal epilepsy induced by massive doses of phenobarbital and midazolam, *Pediatr Neurol*, 51 (2014), 259–61. DOI: https://doi.org/10.1016/j.pediatrneurol.2014.04.004.

121. K. B. Howell, J. M. McMahon, G. L. Carvill et al., SCN2A encephalopathy: a major cause of epilepsy of infancy with migrating focal seizures, *Neurology*, 85 (2015), 958–66. DOI: https://10.1212/WNL.0000000000001926.

122. P. Bittigau, M. Sifringer, C. Ikonomidou, Antiepileptic drugs and apoptosis in the developing brain, *Ann N Y Acad Sci*, 993 (2003), 103–14; discussion 23–4. DOI: https://doi.org/10.1111/j.1749-6632.2003.tb07517.x.

123. A. M. Kaindl, S. Asimiadou, D. Manthey, M. V. Hagen, L. Turski, C. Ikonomidou, Antiepileptic drugs and the developing brain, *Cell Mol*

Life Sci, 63 (2006), 399–413. DOI: https://doi.org/10.1007/s00018-005-5348-0.

124. J. S. Kim, A. Kondratyev, Y. Tomita, K. Gale, Neurodevelopmental impact of antiepileptic drugs and seizures in the immature brain, *Epilepsia*, 48 Suppl 5 (2007), 19–26. DOI: https://doi.org/10.1111/j.1528-1167.2007.01285.x.

125. J. Yanai, F. Fares, M. Gavish et al., Neural and behavioral alterations after early exposure to phenobarbital, *Neurotoxicology*, 10 (1989), 543–54.

126. R. A. Shellhaas, Neonatal seizures reach the mainstream: The ILAE classification of seizures in the neonate, *Epilepsia*, 62 (2021), 629–31. DOI: https://doi.org/10.1111/epi.16857.

127. S. T. Haines, D. T. Casto, Treatment of infantile spasms, *Ann Pharmacother*, 28 (1994), 779–91. DOI: https://doi.org/10.1177/106002809402800616.

128. S. A. Hussain, J. Heesch, J. Weng, R. R. Rajaraman, A. L. Numis, R. Sankar, Potential induction of epileptic spasms by nonselective voltage-gated sodium channel blockade: Interaction with etiology, *Epilepsy Behav*, 115 (2021), 107624. DOI: https://doi.org/10.1016/j.yebeh.2020.107624.

129. P. S. Reif, M. H. Tsai, I. Helbig, F. Rosenow, K. M. Klein, Precision medicine in genetic epilepsies: break of dawn?, *Expert Rev Neurother*, 17 (2017), 381–92. DOI: https://doi.org/10.1080/14737175.2017.1253476.

130. R. M. Pressler, L. Lagae, Why we urgently need improved seizure and epilepsy therapies for children and neonates, *Neuropharmacology*, 170 (2020), 107854. DOI: https://doi.org/10.1016/j.neuropharm.2019.107854.

131. M. Kuersten, M. Tacke, L. Gerstl, H. Hoelz, C. V. Stülpnagel, I. Borggraefe, Antiepileptic therapy approaches in KCNQ2 related epilepsy: A systematic review, *Eur J Med Genet*, 63 (2020), 103628. DOI: https://doi.org/10.1016/j.ejmg.2019.02.001.

132. M. J. Brodie, Sodium channel blockers in the treatment of epilepsy, *CNS Drugs*, 31 (2017), 527–34. DOI: https://doi.org/10.1007/s40263-017-0441-0.

133. Z. Pan, T. Kao, Z. Horvath et al., A common ankyrin-G-based mechanism retains KCNQ and NaV channels at electrically active domains of the axon, *J Neurosci*, 26 (2006), 2599–613. DOI: https://doi.org/10.1523/jneurosci.4314-05.2006.

134. M. Bialer, S. I. Johannessen, M. J. Koepp et al., Progress report on new antiepileptic drugs: a summary of the Fifteenth Eilat Conference on New Antiepileptic Drugs and Devices (EILAT XV). I. Drugs in preclinical and early clinical development, *Epilepsia*, 61 (2020), 2340–64. DOI: https://doi.org/10.1111/epi.16725.

135. I. Premoli, P. G. Rossini, P. Y. Goldberg et al., TMS as a pharmacodynamic indicator of cortical activity of a novel anti-epileptic drug, XEN1101, *Ann Clin Transl Neurol*, 6 (2019), 2164–74. DOI: https://doi.org/10.1002/acn3 .50896.

136. D. Y. Chen, S. Chowdhury, L. Farnaes et al., Rapid diagnosis of KCNQ2-associated early infantile epileptic encephalopathy improved outcome, *Pediatr Neurol*, 86 (2018), 69–70. DOI: https://doi.org/10 .1016/j.pediatrneurol.2018.06.002.

137. Z. Han, C. Chen, A. Christiansen et al., Antisense oligonucleotides increase SCN1A expression and reduce seizures and SUDEP incidence in a mouse model of Dravet syndrome, *Sci Transl Med*, 12 (2020). DOI: https://doi.org/10.1126/scitranslmed.aaz6100.

138. G. M. Lenk, P. Jafar-Nejad, S. F. Hill et al., SCN8A antisense oligonucleo-tide is protective in mouse models of SCN8A encephalopathy and Dravet Syndrome, *Ann Neurol*, 87 (2020), 339–46. DOI: https://doi.org/10.1002/ ana.25676.

139. G. L. Carvill, T. Matheny, J. Hesselberth, S. Demarest, Haploinsufficiency, dominant negative, and gain-of-function mechanisms in epilepsy: matching therapeutic approach to the pathophysiology, *Neurotherapeutics*, 18 (2021), 1500–14. DOI: https://doi.org/10.1007/s13311-021-01137-z.

Acknowledgments

The editors and contributing authors would like to thank Rebecca Oramas for drawing Figures 1, 11 and 12. We also thank Dr. Anne Berg, Stephanie McCormack, Enrique Rojas, and Abbie Van Nuland for providing the infographics from the KCNQ2 natural history study (Figures 2–10). We are grateful to Shaye Moore for proofreading the manuscript and transcribing video interviews.

About the Authors

Sarah Weckhuysen, M.D., Ph.D. is a neurologist at the University Hospital of Antwerp and Assistant Professor of Neurology at the University of Antwerp. She also leads the epilepsy genetics research group at the VIB-Center for Molecular Neurology. Her research has contributed to many different epilepsy gene discoveries, including the demonstration that de novo *KCNQ2* mutations cause a neonatal epileptic encephalopathy.

Alfred L. George, Jr., M.D. is Professor and Chair of Pharmacology at Northwestern University Feinberg School of Medicine. He has been a pioneer in elucidating the genetics and pathogenesis of channelopathies with a focus on genetic disorders caused by voltage-gated ion channel mutations including KCNQ2-associated epilepsy. He directs the Channelopathy-Associated Epilepsy Research Center without Walls funded by the National Institute of Neurological Disorders and Stroke.

Maria Roberta Cilio, M.D., Ph.D. is Professor of Pediatric Neurology at the University of Louvain in Brussels, Belgium, where she serves as a pediatric and neonatal epileptologist at Saint-Luc University Hospital. Her research focuses on the early diagnosis and treatment of seizures and epilepsies in infants. She has demonstrated the efficacy of sodium channel blockers on seizures associated to *KCNQ2* and *KCNQ3*.

Sara James is a renowned broadcast journalist, an advocate for research in epilepsy and community-academic partnerships in genetic epilepsy, and National Strategy Director for the American Chamber of Commerce in Australia. She is Vice President of the KCNQ2 Cure Alliance and a cofounder of Genetic Epilepsy Team Australia.

Caroline Loewy is a biopharmaceutical and financial executive with more than 25 years of experience in the field. She is a cofounder and board member of the KCNQ2 Cure Alliance, supporting research and development of treatments for those, like her son, who are affected by KCNQ2 developmental and epileptic encephalopathy.

Tristan Sands, M.D., Ph.D. is Assistant Professor of Neurology at Columbia University Irving Medical Center in the Division of Child Neurology and the Institute for Genomic Medicine. He is a pediatric and neonatal neurologist and epileptologist with clinical and research focus on epilepsies and developmental and epileptic encephalopathies resulting from *KCNQ2* and *KCNQ3*.

Scotty Sims is a crisis therapist who provides support and assessment to children and adults with severe and persistent mental illness. After her daughter was diagnosed with *KCNQ2* encephalopathy, she started an international KCNQ2 parent support group for families struggling with a diagnosis of KCNQ2 developmental and epileptic encephalopathy.

Maurizio Taglialatela, M.D., Ph.D. is Professor of Pharmacology at the University of Naples Federico II in Naples, Italy. His research on voltage-gated potassium channels including KCNQ2 and KCNQ3 has revealed import-ant mechanisms responsible for channel function, pharmacology and the func-tional consequences of pathogenic variants associated with epilepsy and other phenotypes of the KCNQ2- and KCNQ3-related disorders spectrum.

Tammy N. Tsuchida, M.D., Ph.D. is a neurophysiologist and neonatal neurolo-gist at Children's National Hospital, and Professor of Neurology and Pediatrics at the George Washington University School of Medicine and Health Sciences. She has expertise in the diagnosis and treatment of childhood epilepsy including disorders associated with *KCNQ2* and *KCNQ3*.

Anastasios Tzingounis, Ph.D. is Professor of Physiology and Neurobiology at the University of Connecticut. His research has contributed to elucidating mechanisms by which epilepsy-associated molecules and signaling networks lead to epileptogenesis in the neonatal and infantile brain. He has made import-ant discoveries about the neurophysiology of *KCNQ2*- and *KCNQ3*-associated epilepsy using genetically engineered mice.

Cambridge Elements ☰

Genetics in Epilepsy

Editor in Chief
Annapurna H. Poduri
Boston Children's Hospital and Harvard Medical School

Annapurna H. Poduri, M.D., MPH is Professor of Neurology at Harvard Medical School. She is Director of the Epilepsy Genetics Program at Boston Children's Hospital, which focuses on the discovery of germline and mosaic variants in patients with epilepsy, and modeling epilepsy genes in zebrafish and cell-based models.

Deputy Editors
Alfred L. George, Jr.
Northwestern University Feinberg School of Medicine

Alfred L. George, Jr., M.D. is Professor and Chair of Pharmacology at the Northwestern University Feinberg School of Medicine. He directs the Channelopathy-associated Epilepsy Research Center without Walls, supported by the National Institutes of Neurological Disorders and Stroke, connecting patient variants with bench science.

Erin L. Heinzen
University of North Carolina, Chapel Hill

Erin L. Heinzen, Pharm.D., Ph.D. is Associate Professor of Pharmacy and Genetics at the University of North Carolina at Chapel Hill. She has served as Principal Investigator of the Sequencing, Biostatistics & Bioinformatics Core of the Epi4K Consortium and investigates somatic mosaic mutation in epilepsy and the mechanisms underlying SLC35A2 epilepsy.

Associate Editor
Sara James
KCNQ2 Cure Alliance and Genetic Epilepsy Team Australia

Sara James is a renowned broadcast journalist and an advocate for research in epilepsy and community-academic partnerships in genetic epilepsy. She is Vice President of the KCNQ2 Cure Alliance and a cofounder of Genetic Epilepsy Team Australia

About the Series
Recent advances in epilepsy genetics are actively revealing numerous genetic contributors to epilepsy, both inherited and noninherited, collectively accounting for a substantial portion of otherwise unexplained epilepsies. This series integrates clinical epilepsy genetics and laboratory research, driving the field toward more precise and effective treatments.

Cambridge Elements ≡

Genetics in Epilepsy

Elements in the Series

12 301

Printed by Printforce, the Netherlands